NURTURE YOUR BODY

OVERCOMING AND PREVENTING OBESITY

CARMEL D. BROWN

ARNICA PRESS

Published by ARNICA PRESS
www.ArnicaPress.com

Cover photo by Stockcreations

ISBN: 978-1-7352446-3-1

NURTURE YOUR BODY

OVERCOMING AND PREVENTING OBESITY

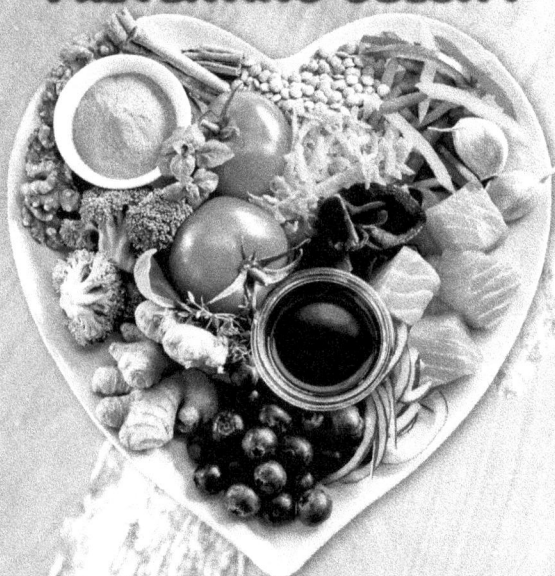

CARMEL D. BROWN

I dedicate this book to my mother,
who has continued to push me,
support me, and cheer me on throughout my life.
Thanks for being a great mother and a great friend.
Thanks for being a mother with high expectations,
correcting me when I needed to be corrected,
and teaching me what hard work is.
You have been an excellent role model for our family.
I love you, Mom!

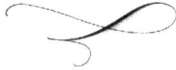

TABLE OF CONTENTS

ACKNOWLEDGMENTS

I would like to acknowledge my family and friends
who continue to support me, encourage me,
and pray for me.

I would like to give a huge acknowledgment
to my husband, Rodney.

Thanks for being my rock, constantly encouraging me,
and for being the love of my life
and my best friend.

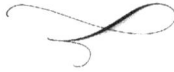

INTRODUCTION

This book was written to give individuals who are absolute beginners a guide to follow when deciding to lose weight, improve their emotional and physical health, and to live an overall healthy lifestyle.

There are new trends in health and fitness, new and ongoing studies on health and fitness, numerous health and fitness magazines on the stands, numerous fitness centers, many health and fitness shows on television, various authors on health and fitness, many internet fitness channels and/or professionals, and so on. It can become quite overwhelming at times, especially when you hear or read conflicting information.

Each individual has to find a starting point, regimen, or program that works best for him or her in order to succeed at living a healthier lifestyle.

Yesterday you said you would start tomorrow.
Today is tomorrow,
so make it happen today!

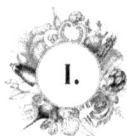

Chapter I.
The Obesity Crisis

Since the early twentieth century, Americans have nearly doubled our meat consumption, more than tripled our sugar consumption, and more than doubled our dairy products consumption annually. Researchers estimate that these increases have been a major factor in the obesity epidemic our nation faces today. Our food supply contains excessive amounts of preservatives, additives, hormones, and steroids. Many researchers and health professionals believe this has contributed to health conditions such as obesity, diabetes, heart disease, hypertension, severe allergies, cancer, and many other diseases. Today more than one third of US adults are overweight, one third are obese, and one third are in the normal or healthy-weight range. Public Health officials estimate that obesity rates for children have doubled over the past few decades. The *American Journal of Preventative Medicine* released a study in 2012 predicting that 42 percent of Americans will be obese by 2030. After examining data from 1990 to 2008, researchers predicted that the obesity rate will increase by one third and that the rate of severe obesity in the United States will jump by more than 100 percent over the next two decades. If this increase occurs, millions of Americans will have major health problems, which will result in over $500 billion in health-care costs.

After eating an excessive amount of calories decades ago, most Americans walked, worked, and engaged in activities in which they burned calories. In addition, Americans did not drive everywhere, and food wasn't as processed or convenient as it is today. In some cases, physical activity was required in order to acquire food such as fishing, hunting, farming, gardening, and so forth.

Today all we have to do is pick up the phone and order or pull up to a drive-thru. Convenience is literally killing us! The days of having to go out to hunt for your food or grow and raise your own food are far behind us. Obviously, we still have local farmers and the larger suppliers of meat, dairy, and produce, but most Americans no longer have family members with farms and gardens. Throughout my childhood my paternal and maternal grandparents had gardens with fresh produce. I believe this made a difference in the type of food we became accustomed to snacking on. I remember snacking on carrots, cucumbers, and tomatoes regularly as a child. Obesity did not become problematic to our society until the mid-twentieth century, when convenience food and TV dinners became popular. A large portion of the food we consume is unhealthy and/or unsafe since it is processed, contains chemicals and hormones, and is prepared with numerous artificial ingredients. Due to convenience, we are exerting very little physical activity before or after we eat. A constant and ongoing surplus of calories for most Americans also contributes to our widespread obesity epidemic. Excessive calorie consumption occurs daily; however, the daily physical activity needed to burn off those calories is not performed by most people. If we were less sedentary, like Americans were decades ago, our bodies would burn the extra energy or calories stored from the previous day, reducing the risk of storing extra calories as fat. This would reduce the occurrence of obesity and obesity-related illnesses.

Genetics play a major role in the obesity epidemic we face today. According to the Centers for Disease Control (CDC), genes give the body instructions for responding to changes in its environment. Studies of resemblances and differences among family members, twins, and adopted children offer indirect scientific evidence that a significant portion of the variation in weight among adults is due to genetic factors. Other studies have compared obese and nonobese people for variation in genes that could influence behaviors such as a drive or tendency to overeat, a tendency to be sedentary, or metabolism (such as a diminished capacity to use dietary fats as fuel or an increased tendency to store body fat). These studies have identified variants in several genes that may contribute to obesity by increasing hunger and food intake. Usually there is no clear pattern of inherited obesity within a family that is caused by a specific variant of a single gene (monogenic obesity). Most cases of obesity are possibly the result of complex interactions among multiple genes, and environmental factors that we still don't understand (multifactorial obesity). There is still a significant amount of research that needs to be conducted in this area.

> *Although there is evidence*
> *that genetic predisposition to obesity exists,*
> *a healthy lifestyle can counteract this predisposition.*

Let's break that down in simple terms. A person born into a family in which obesity is common and/or prevalent is at high risk for being obese. You may have noticed families in the shopping mall or grocery store in which both parents and the children were overweight. I could use my family for example. Many of the women in my family are overweight. Most of them were at a healthy Body Mass Index prior to having children or when they were younger. I gained 52 pounds with my first pregnancy, and another 45 pounds with my second pregnancy. This was an indication that my body has no problem packing on large amounts of weight. I have worked very hard at living a healthy lifestyle over the years in order to avoid obesity. If I had not maintained a healthy lifestyle, I would have held onto the extra 97 pounds I gained from the 2 pregnancies.

Genetic predisposition also applies to individuals with a lean build. We have all met that person that doesn't exercise, has no restrictions on what they will eat or how much, and manages to maintain a lean body. I remember meeting a very slender young lady in our gym who'd given birth to five children. I was shocked when she disclosed she was the mother of five children, but not as shocked as I was when she told me she was an absolute beginner at fitness. Because she was very thin I assumed she exercised at least semi-regularly. This told me that genetically she was not predisposed to obesity as I am. Typically a lean body is an indication of good health, and an overweight body is an indicator of poor health. However, this isn't always the case for various reasons. Unhealthy habits such as substance abuse, various medical conditions, or chronic illness can result in poor nutrition or malnutrition, and low body weight. Unfortunately, in cases such as these, a thin build may suggest poor health.

Today we have more diet products and programs guaranteed to make you lose weight than ever. However our obesity epidemic in the United States keeps getting worse. Let's take a closer look at some of the previously mentioned contributing factors to the rapid growth of the obesity crisis in the United States such as:

1. Food supply is not as safe or nutritious as it once was
2. Lack of physical activity & exercise
3. Poor diet
4. Lack of education regarding nutrition
5. Poor metabolism

1. Food supply

Our food supply is not as healthy as it was decades ago. In the 1950s a regular fast-food burger was less than three ounces and barely over two hundred calories. Today that same burger is more than four ounces and more than three hundred calories. A regular cola soda grew from six ounces in the early twentieth to twenty ounces in the late 1990s. In addition, we now have access to numerous sodas and beverages containing over forty ounces of chemicals, sugar, and carbonation in most gas stations and restaurants. Americans who struggle with obesity, fast-food addiction, or sugar addiction have unlimited access to many of their "drugs of choice" on every corner, at restaurants, convenience stores, and gas stations.

Another factor affecting the quality of our food supply is that some of the meat we consume contains dangerous levels of hormones, antibiotics, and steroids and sometimes comes from different countries or unknown sources. Grocers are now required to indicate the country in which our meat is shipped from on packaging.

Since our meat comes from unknown and sometimes harmful sources there are an estimated 3,000 annual deaths and over 130,000 hospitalizations due to foodborne illness. Although this is tragic, it is fairly minor compared to other deaths related to our diet. Each year more than 300,000 Americans die earlier than necessary, and many more are sick due to largely preventable, diet-related conditions. These conditions include heart disease, diabetes, obesity, hypertension, strokes, and some cancers.

The biggest problem with our food supply isn't just pathogens. Our biggest problem is processed food. We're not being killed by *E.*

coli and *Salmonella*, but by the nutrient-poor contents of the bags, boxes, and fast food that we consume daily. About 70 percent of the calories Americans consume today come from highly processed foods loaded with salt, sugar, fat, unfamiliar additives, and refined grains that have been stripped of naturally occurring nutrients and antioxidants. We've outsourced too much of our cooking and meal preparation to convenient food companies that prepare meals very differently than we do in our homes.

2. LACK OF PHYSICAL ACTIVITY & EXERCISE

Lack of physical activity is also a contributing factor to the obesity crisis in the United States. Several occupations have been identified as being linked to a high risk of obesity. These occupations include but are not limited to truck drivers, transit drivers, and people who sit at a desk and/or computer all day with little to no movement. Construction workers, health diagnosing occupations, postsecondary teachers, and food preparation workers seem to have the lowest incidence of obesity. Each of us has unique and individual needs and circumstances that may be contributing to weight or health problems, but the good news is no one is sentenced to an irreversible or permanent life of obesity. Thyroid problems, various medications, pregnancy, and genetics can contribute to weight gain, but ultimately the aforementioned conditions and circumstances are not the cause of our long-term weight problem as a nation—they are simply contributing factors.

Schools all over the country are experiencing budget cuts, which has negatively affected physical education programs in many school districts. The CDC recommends that children ages six to seventeen get sixty minutes of aerobic exercise daily at a moderate to vigorous intensity level. This should include strength-building exercises such as push-ups and sit-ups, and bone-building exercises such as jumping rope, and climbing stairs. If you believe your children need more exercise or don't meet these recommendations contact your local YMCA, community center, or other fitness centers to enroll your children in weekly programming to keep them active. I encourage parents to get outside with their children to walk, jog, ride bikes, swim, hike, or engage in some type of weekly activities that promote an active lifestyle.

The CDC recommends that adults ages eighteen to sixty-four get 150 minutes (or two and a half hours) of aerobic exercise weekly at moderate intensity. This should include strength training on at least two days each week. If aerobic exercise is performed at vigorous intensity, one hour and fifteen minutes per week is considered sufficient. For older adults age sixty-five and older, the CDC recommends two and a half hours of moderate exercise weekly or one and a half hours of vigorous exercise. This should include two days of strength or resistance training such as weight lifting.

3. POOR DIET

Many Americans have a poor diet simply because we like convenience, most of us choose food based on flavor rather than nutrition, and we are busier than ever! In most households both parents work outside of the home, and most children are involved in several extracurricular activities outside of the home. The busy life that most Americans live leaves very little down time to prepare a menu for the week, and cook three well-balanced meals each day. The cost of living continues to rise, and it has become more difficult to budget on one income, and still live comfortably for many families. Since no one has time to cook, most families are eating fast food or unhealthy processed food for the sake of saving time and money.

When this pattern continues over a long period of time, it becomes unhealthy and results in poor health. It costs three to five dollars to get a meal from a fast-food chain, and it takes less than ten minutes for them to prepare your food. It is much more time consuming to cook a healthy meal at home and, in some cases, more expensive if you are trying to stick to healthy, whole foods. It takes a lot of planning and preparation to avoid the unhealthy pattern or routine that most of us busy American families find ourselves in. We have an extensive long list of lifestyle changes to make in order to improve our current obesity crisis in the United States.

4. LACK OF EDUCATION REGARDING NUTRITION

We have failed to properly educate our communities and families on proper nutrition, such as which foods are essential for preventing or contributing to weight loss, which foods are essential for overall health, nutritional value of food, and how to read nutrition labels on food. It is imperative that we understand why we should incorporate certain foods into our diet and which foods we should remove from our diet. This book will provide insight in both areas.

5. POOR METABOLISM

Metabolism is another contributing factor to the obesity crisis. However, it is not as much of a contributing factor as the four aforementioned concerns, thereforeso it will be discussed in detail in later chapters.

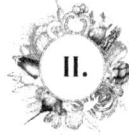

CHAPTER II.
BATTLING OBESITY

Daily exercise, proper nutrition, adequate rest, reduced stress, healthy metabolism, and hydration combined will have the most significant impact on weight loss or weight gain. I have trained several clients who had poor diets but weren't gaining weight because they were burning a lot of calories during their training sessions. However, they weren't losing the weight they were trying so hard to lose due to poor diet, poor sleep habits, insufficient hydration throughout the day, excessive cortisol levels due to ongoing and chronic stress, or some combination of the listed circumstances. This results in frustration and affects their level of motivation since people don't see any movement on the scale or changes in their bodies. As previously stated, the number on the scale isn't the only indicator of progress, but spending hundreds of dollars and multiple hours training each week for months at a time with little or no results can be very discouraging.

Many people blame their weight gain or failure in the battle against obesity on slow metabolism. Most people don't understand how metabolism works or what it is, so let's go through a brief description and explanation of how it works, and why it is relevant in the battle against obesity.

> *Metabolism is the process of converting what you eat and drink into energy.*

During this process, calories in food and beverages are combined with oxygen to release the energy your body needs to function.

It's true that metabolism is linked to our weight, and it slows down as we get older, but slow metabolism is usually not the actual cause of weight gain or obesity. Your body's energy requirements to process food stay relatively steady and aren't easily changed.

When you're at rest, your body still needs energy for all of its normal functions like circulating blood, adjusting hormone levels, breathing, and so forth. The number of calories your body uses to carry out these basic functions is known as your basal metabolic rate. On average basal metabolic rate accounts for around 70 percent of the calories you burn every day for most individuals. Being aware of this information can help understand how basic bodily functions impacts our waistline.

Physical activity and exercise account for the rest of the calories your body burns each day. Physical activity is by far the most variable of the factors that determine how many calories you burn each day, since our activity level, type of activity, and duration of activity vary from day to day.

Many weight-loss programs are not successful in helping clients win the battle against obesity, or they work only in the short-term because they either promote a healthy diet without providing a consistent training schedule or focus on training without addressing nutrition. Many Americans attempt to lose weight by following a very-low-calorie diet (VLCD), or crash/fad diets. Strict dieting can have a negative impact on metabolism, which affects your body's ability to burn calories consumed. Any diet that suggests eating fewer than twelve hundred calories daily will typically leave you hungry, tired, deprived, grumpy, and outright miserable. The only time such extreme dieting is safe is when prescribed by a physician and is medically supervised.

> *Both exercise and a healthy-meal plan*
> *are necessary for long-term success.*

As a trainer, I hate to admit that you can lose weight without exercise. However, I don't recommend leaving exercise out of the equation for several reasons. People who exercise live longer, have a stronger heart, less risk of depression, a lower percentage of body fat, reduced stress, higher self-esteem, less risk of diseases like diabetes, and even manage symptoms of mental illness better. It makes more sense to be at a healthy weight with improved physical and mental health rather than just being at a healthy weight. Being able to fit in your skinny jeans while unhealthy, chronically fatigued, in a bad mood, and sick is pretty pointless. It is a better idea to lose weight in a healthy manner so that you can enjoy life and enjoy your results. It is important to maintain a well-balanced diet and exercise regularly to achieve and maintain your results.

One of the most basic concepts to keep in mind with your weight-loss efforts is "calories in, calories out." If you eat more calories than you burn each day, you will more than likely gain weight. If you burn more calories than you eat, it is highly likely you will lose weight, and at the very minimum you will maintain your current weight. It should be noted that there are exceptions to every rule, so not everyone who follows this basic principle will lose weight. There are various medical conditions, certain medications, and other circumstances that could hinder weight loss. Not all calories are created equal, therefore the quality of the food you eat is just as important as burning the calories you consume.

Eating four to six times a day is also a proven, effective strategy for weight loss. Eating smaller meals more frequently prevents feelings of deprivation, keeps us energized during exercise, helps control blood sugar and insulin, boosts metabolism, establishes a regular pattern of eating, and helps prevent impulse eating. Your daily meal plan should include breakfast, lunch, dinner, and one or two snacks. You are less likely to binge if you eat throughout the day. It is very easy to exceed your daily recommended caloric intake when eating four to six times a day, so tracking calories and macronutrients in the beginning is important. Most meals should be small, keeping breakfast, lunch, and dinner to three hundred to four hundred calories each and snacks at one hundred calories or less (based on an individual weighing less than 160 lbs. with a daily caloric goal of twelve hundred to fifteen hundred calories).

An individual weighing less than 160 pounds should consume about twelve hundred to fifteen hundred calories each day for weight loss. Your level of activity and individual fitness goals will have to be taken into consideration to pinpoint an exact number of recommended calories.

An individual weighing between 160 and 300 pounds should multiply their weight by seven to get an estimated daily calorie goal. For example, if you weigh 200 pounds, multiplying by seven gives fourteen hundred calories, so a range of fourteen hundred to seventeen hundred calories each day is your goal. If you weigh more than 300 pounds, try eating around twenty-one hundred to twenty-two hundred calories each day.

These daily caloric recommendations are to be used as a guide only and will vary from person to person based on numerous factors. It is important to remember that everyone has different nutritional needs based on medical status, goals, height, weight, and activity level.

> *Consult with your physician prior to starting*
> *any physical-fitness program or nutritional program,*
> *especially if you have been diagnosed*
> *with any medical condition,*
> *have dietary restrictions,*
> *or have any concerns about your health.*

As I mentioned earlier, counting calories is not as important as the type of food and the quality of food you eat. Remember, not all calories are created equal, so try to fill your diet with fresh fruits and vegetables, lean meats, whole grains, and healthy fats. If you are eating processed food (packaged, frozen, or canned) with lots of preservatives, trans fats, sugar, and sodium, you are robbing your body of the nutrition it needs to function and perform optimally.

When choosing snacks, go for filling foods containing protein and/or fiber. It doesn't matter that your small package of cookies contains only one hundred calories if the cookies are of poor nutritional value. You will feel much more satisfied after eating an eighty-calorie apple than you will after eating a one-hundred-calorie package of cookies due to the apple's superior nutritional value.

Meals should be balanced, and nutrient dense. I recommend eating fresh vegetables, whole grains, and lean protein containing three to five hundred calories (depending on your daily calorie goal) over a processed or frozen meal containing fewer calories. Most frozen meals contain excessive sodium and unhealthy artificial ingredients. Consumers tend to be fooled by the number of calories in many of these meals. Although one of these frozen meals might have less than 300 calories, most of them have very little nutritional value. Fish, chicken, turkey, broccoli, spinach, asparagus, salad, fruit, water, green tea, and nuts may not be the most exciting daily diet, but feeling good in your own skin, having loads of energy, sleeping well at night, and being able to wear the clothes you desire to wear are all very exciting.

In order to succeed at battling obesity, you have to change your relationship with food and acknowledge the purpose food is supposed to serve in your life. If you fail to do so, it will be extremely difficult to meet your fitness and weight-loss goals.

> *Food is to be used as nourishment and energy and nothing more.*

Somehow as a nation we have started to use overeating as a sport (try tennis or kickball for a sport instead), a leisure time activity (try walking or reading a book) and a way to satisfy our emotions (try counseling or meditation instead). Just turn on your television any day of the week and count the number of television shows based on food, cooking, and/or overeating. There are many popular TV shows based on competitive eating on which contestants compete to see who can eat the most. Eating excessively for pleasure has become very popular in the United States. The outcome is we are engaging in self-harming behavior as any addict of any other substance would do. If food consumption results in deterioration in health but you still can't seem to get your portions under control, it is possible that food has become an addiction and that you require professional help. Seeking help from a certified fitness and nutrition specialist, registered dietitian, physician, or in some cases a licensed therapist would be a great start.

> *We have to be intentional*
> *about making it a priority to remain educated*
> *on facts regarding health and nutrition*
> *otherwise, we put ourselves and our families*
> *at risk for obesity.*

As in most cases, knowledge is key. Being knowledgeable or familiar with ingredients listed on the packaging of foods we eat is a significant part of being educated on our food supply. If we are unaware or unfamiliar with the ingredient list on our food, our families are at an increased risk for ingesting chemicals and additives that can make us sick and overweight.

Becoming familiar with macronutrient requirements is also important for people who desire to improve their health and/or lose weight. Macronutrients are nutrients such as protein, carbohydrates, and fats that the human body needs in large amounts from our diet. Macronutrients are the only sources of energy. I often observe clients count calories vs. counting chemicals and macronutrients. Although being aware of whether we are consuming more or less calories than we need is very beneficial when trying to lose weight or gain weight, being able to manage portions, being aware of whether the ingredients in our food are harmful, and ensuring we are including enough macronutrients in our diet are equally important. Becoming knowledgeable regarding which foods contain these macronutrients, pairing the right foods together, and ensuring we are getting enough of these nutrients are all important in maintaining a well-balanced diet and achieving our health and fitness goals.

Let's first discuss Carbohydrates. Carbohydrates are macronutrients that consist of the starches we find in grains, legumes/beans, vegetables, and fruits. We get some carbohydrates from dairy products but almost none from meats. Our bodies convert most carbohydrates to glucose, which provides a source of energy for cells and tissue. When most people think of carbohydrates they think of bread, pasta, and rice. Many people don't realize our fruits and vegetables fall into the category of carbohydrates, and many people view carbohydrates as unhealthy. The Institute of Medicine and the National Academy of Sports Medicine recommends that 45–65 percent of our total caloric intake consist of carbohydrates. There is no need to reduce carbohydrate intake in order to reduce percentage of body fat, but being choosy about the source or type of carbohydrates we eat and controlling our portions of carbohydrates are both necessary to lose fat. When consuming carbs, remember that each gram of carbohydrates yields four calories, so if your plate of steamed vegetables has twenty grams of carbohydrates that would equal eighty calories. Excessive intake of carbohydrates is not what is making our nation overweight. As a nation, we continue to try fad diets and quick fixes, regardless of how many times we have failed or gained the weight back. Instead of yo-yo dieting, we have to exercise the patience and take the time to learn how to plan, develop, and follow a well-balanced diet with a variety of foods. Liquid diets, starvation diets, and very-low-calorie diets might help lose weight temporarily, but it is highly unlikely that you will keep the weight off. In most cases people not only gain the weight back but end up weighing more than they did before they lost weight. Each time we gain the weight back, we find it more difficult to lose it again. This cycle of extreme dieting is unhealthy and does not produce long-lasting results. I have never met a person who has experienced long-term success from fad diets. Anyone who does experience success with extreme dieting has very little chance of being happy or healthy while doing so.

> *Numerous studies have shown*
> *that an insufficient amount of sleep*
> *is linked to the risk of obesity.*

Most Americans are unaware of the link between sleep deprivation and obesity. The less time a person sleeps, the more time they have for eating. Sleep duration also affects leptin and ghrelin, hormones that regulate hunger. Lack of sleep increases the release of the hormone ghrelin, an appetite stimulant referred to as the hunger hormone, which makes us want to eat more. Lack of sleep also reduces the release of leptin, the hormone that makes us want to eat less. Poor sleep habits also lead to fatigue, which naturally results in less physical activity. In most studies sleeping less than five hours but also more than nine hours a night appears to increase the likelihood of weight gain. According to Dr. Timothy Morgenthaler and Mayo Clinic, infants and toddlers need nine to ten hours of sleep each night (plus two or three naps during the day), adults need seven to eight hours of sleep, and school-aged children need nine to eleven hours of sleep each night.

The Mayo Clinic reports recurrent sleep deprivation in men increased their preferences for high-calorie foods and a higher overall calorie intake. In another study, women who slept less than six hours a night or more than nine hours were more likely to gain ten or more pounds compared with women who slept seven to nine hours a night. Other studies have found similar patterns in children and adolescents.

> *Educating ourselves and our communities*
> *on the proper strategies for assessing*
> *our health and fitness status*
> *is also important in the fight against obesity.*

This includes refraining from relying on your bathroom scale to tell you the entire story regarding your health and knowing which professionals can help with assessments, treatment, and training.

Body mass index (BMI) measures the proportion of weight to height, and remains the most widely used marker of obesity around the world. The difference between being considered obese and overweight is significant. A person who is considered obese has a BMI of more than thirty, compared to a person who is overweight with a BMI of 25.0 to 30.0. A normal BMI is between the 18.5 and 24.9. Anything under 18.5 is considered underweight.

There are numerous limitations when using Body Mass Index calculations as a method of measuring good health. A good example of the limitations would be a body builder or athlete with a very low body-fat percentage who gains fifteen pounds of lean muscle. If this extra fifteen pounds of lean muscle mass results in the individual exceeding the recommended weight for their height, the BMI calculator would indicate this person is overweight. BMI calculations do not take into consideration the difference between fat and muscle - BMI simply calculates the extra pounds as excess weight. This is frustrating for someone who has a lower body-fat percentage and a better physique than someone of the same height with a higher percentage of body fat and lower weight. BMI calculations would suggest the person with the higher body-fat percentage is in better health because they weigh less at the same height.

Measuring body-fat percentage is a much better indicator of overall health compared to BMI. Skinfold measurements, circumference measurements, and bioelectrical impedance are all good methods for measuring body-fat percentage. Underwater weighing or hydrostatic weighing is another method of assessing body-fat percentage and has been proven to be very accurate. Hydrostatic weighing is most commonly used in exercise physiology labs, so your local fitness center is unlikely to have this as an option for determining body composition.

Waist-to-hip ratio is also a very effective assessment that indicates an individual's overall risk for disease. This entails measuring hips and waist and assessing risk for disease. A certified personal trainer can help measure the waist-to-hip ratio.

Fat is more or less of a health risk depending on where it is stored. For example, fat in the hip and/or thigh area is far less dangerous than abdominal fat or organ fat, which increases the risk of insulin resistance and diabetes. The assessments and methods of measuring body fat listed in this chapter will help understand potential health risks based on your body composition and body fat percentage.

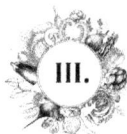

CHAPTER III.
BATTLING CRAVINGS

Many people who are overweight have ongoing cravings and poor metabolism due to history of crash dieting and binge eating. It is important to note that the brain also has some impact on cravings. The same areas of our brain that are responsible for memory and sensing pleasure are partially to blame for food cravings.

Filling up on foods that are packed with water and fiber are a great approach to remaining full between meals, hence reducing cravings. Many Americans find that they are hungry, moody, and experiencing extreme and uncontrollable cravings throughout their day. This is partially due to today's processed food being loaded with calories, sugar, and fat rather than dense and filling nutrition. This affects the brain's reward center and drives us to overeat.

According to scientists using brain-imaging technology at the National Institutes of Health, when large amounts of fat, sugar, and calories are consumed, you get the same brain response seen in individuals addicted to heroin.

According to scientists using brain-imaging technology at the National Institutes of Health, when large amounts of fat sugar, and calories are consumed, you get the same brain response seen in individuals addicted to heroin. This is an indication that food addiction truly does exist. When you start to eat more whole foods rather than processed foods, the cravings automatically start to diminish. Transitioning to a more nutrient-dense diet will result in improved mental clarity (no more brain fog), increased energy, improved sleep patterns, better performance of your body, increased energy and power for your workouts, and an increased likelihood of achieving your weight-loss goals. Moreover, you will experience an overall improved quality of life.

One proven effective strategy for battling cravings is drinking a glass or two of water to make sure you aren't mistaking thirst for hunger. If you are still hungry after drinking a glass of water, enjoy a small snack that includes a little protein such as a boiled egg (try to go with whites only if possible), low-fat Greek yogurt, or a handful of nuts.

Remove all trigger foods, such as items containing high-fructose corn syrup (HFCS), trans fats, sugar listed as one of the first three ingredients, or that include ingredients that you can't pronounce or you are unfamiliar with. Get rid of all packaged foods that are loaded with artificial ingredients, preservatives, and large amounts of sodium, as these items result in extreme cravings when eaten. Reducing stress is also a good way to battle cravings, especially if you tend to eat or snack mindlessly when emotionally overwhelmed. Positive thinking, positive self-talk, prayer, meditation, a massage, watching comedy on television, and a great playlist with your favorite tunes are all great ways to relax. If you find that stress is a constant problem and is interfering with your quality of life, consult a licensed therapist to discuss coping skills and activities to manage ongoing stress.

When you fail to plan and prepare you typically find yourself famished. Extreme hunger typically results in unstable blood sugar, cravings, unhealthy snacking, and binge eating. For these reasons, it is important to plan and prepare snacks and meals in advance. Try keeping it simple to salads, wraps, combination bowls (for example, quinoa or beans, avocado, chicken or shrimp, kale or spinach, edamame mixed in a bowl). You can add salsa, a dash of hot pepper sauce, or low-sodium teriyaki sauce if you need to add flavor. Keeping it simple rather than planning and prepping elaborate meals and snacks makes it easier to maintain healthy habits long-term. In addition, prepping meals that require several ingredients can be time consuming, expensive, and outright overwhelming. Lean protein, healthy fats, and complex carbs will help remain satisfied between meals, therefore you will experience fewer cravings.

> *If you still find it impossible to battle excessive cravings after implementing the aforementioned strategies, consider speaking to your doctor or a professional therapist about an assessment to determine if there is a problem that requires medication or additional treatment.*

Sometimes stress and poor coping skills can result in excessive snacking. A physician can prescribe medication if necessary, and a therapist can help acquire healthy coping skills that won't result in weight gain and deterioration of health.

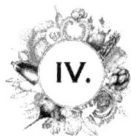

CHAPTER IV.
THE F.. WORD

Today we know more than ever about body fat and dietary fat, and how they affect each other. We are all born with a specific number of fat cells. The average person has about ten to twenty billion fat cells in his or her body. Scientists who study obesity believe that throughout life we retain the same number of fat cells we are born with. However, the amount of fat inside of the cells or the size of our fat cells changes as we lose and gain weight. Researchers in Sweden report that 10 percent of our fat cells die each year and those cells are replaced with new fat cells.

> *When calories are consumed in excess,*
> *our bodies store the excess calories as fat.*

The best way to prevent increases in body-fat percentage is to follow a balanced diet filled with fruits, vegetables, lean protein, low-fat dairy, whole grains, remaining hydrated, adequate sleep, and daily exercise.

In the past, many Americans have refrained from eating dietary fats due to fat's bad reputation. For years fat was viewed as unhealthy and something to be avoided, a nonessential, undesirable part of the American diet. During those years Americans were obsessed with low-fat diets, and we found and increase of low-fat versions of food on the shelves in our grocery stores. Since then we have found that fat is necessary in order for the body to perform optimally. Research has proven the human body needs fat to function, fats are essential in the absorption of vitamins A, D, and E, and fats are vital for our nervous system. The type of fat we consume and the portion/ amount of fats we consume are key. For example, many of our packaged and processed foods contain trans fats, which is a type of fat that should never be consumed. The FDA has declared trans fats unsafe due to linkage to coronary heart disease. We typically find trans fats in foods such as crackers, cookies, cakes, microwave popcorn, frozen pies, stick margarine, coffee creamers, refrigerated dough products, and frostings.

Monounsaturated and polyunsaturated fats such as those found in avocados, nuts, olives, some oils, salmon, and cold-water fish have numerous health benefits. Monounsaturated fatty acids found in cold-water fish, such as salmon, have favorable effects on helping to prevent heart disease, cancer, hypertension, and arthritis. This type of fat is considered healthy and raise our HDL, or good cholesterol, and lower our LDL, or bad cholesterol. Although monounsaturated fats are the healthiest type of fat, I still caution you simply because even healthy sources of fat can be high in calories.

Polyunsaturated fatty acids provide very important essential fatty acids that can't be produced or manufactured by the body, but are essential for proper health and functioning. Since the human body can't make omega-3 or omega-6 fatty acids, we must get them through food or a supplement. Polyunsaturated fats contain essential fatty acids and positively affect cholesterol, improve brain function, strengthen the immune system, and improve our mood. Omega-6 fatty acids can help keep our skin and eyes healthy. You will find omega-3's primarily in fish such as salmon, mackerel, and herring. You will also find omega-3 fatty acids in canola oil, flaxseed, walnuts, and tofu. Both omega-3 and omega-6 fatty acids play a major role in brain function, growth, and development. Omega-6 fatty acids are found in safflower oil, corn oil, corn-fed chicken and beef, and farm-raised fish.

Excessive amounts of omega-6 fatty acids can be a risk to our health by putting us at risk for high blood pressure, heart disease, stroke, and blood clots. If you have not already, it's time to get rid of vegetable oil, shortening, and all unhealthy fats. Trade them in for olive oil, raw organic coconut oil, and canola oil when possible.

> *Saturated fats are not what I consider*
> *a healthy source of fat since they have*
> *the potential to raise cholesterol levels*
> *and increase your risk of heart disease.*

Saturated fats are found in meat and poultry, dairy products, butter, and in a few plant-based foods such as palm oil. Saturated fat is usually solid at room temperature. One easy way to reduce saturated-fat intake is to remove the skin from your meat. Although saturated fats are not the healthiest type of fat, recent studies are suggesting saturated fats are not as bad for us as we previously believed.

There has been a lot of controversy surrounding coconut oil and whether it is good for you. Coconut oil is a saturated fat, but we must acknowledge recent findings from the medical community on the benefits of coconut oil. It may increase healthy cholesterol (HDL), and help convert bad cholesterol (LDL) into good cholesterol.

Researchers believe coconut oil promotes heart health and reduces the risk of heart disease. It also helps absorb other nutrients such as vitamins, minerals, and amino acids. Coconut oil also has many antimicrobial properties in helping to deal with bacteria, fungus, and so forth. When purchasing coconut oil, be sure to get the unrefined virgin oil, and keep daily use to a minimum. As with other types of fat, serving size is important.

Fat does not make you fat.
Sugar, refined and processed food,
taking in more calories than you burn daily,
inadequate sleep, lack of hydration,
not eating enough calories or the right type of foods,
and various medical conditions
contribute to obesity.

A fat-free diet is no longer popular, nor is it a good choice. Choosing healthy sources of fat is key in helping our bodies function properly. Healthy fats reduce the risk of metabolic syndrome, reduce inflammation, reduce the risk of breast cancer, improve brain health, target belly fat, and promote longevity. In addition, fat triggers the release of antihunger hormones and improves the absorption of vitamin D, which is known to speed weight loss.

Avocados, one of my favorite monounsaturated fats, can easily be over two hundred calories and twenty grams of fat for one avocado. You have to be mindful of your portion sizes with fats. Use one-fourth of an avocado for meals, which typically adds less than sixty calories and about five grams of fat.

Peanut butter and almond butter are great sources of fat as well but are often overused and abused. Just one tablespoon of peanut butter can be around ninety-five calories and eight grams of fat. When possible use the natural versions of peanut butter, and read the ingredients to ensure there aren't a lot of added ingredients such as sugar and salt. All it takes to make peanut butter is peanuts and oil, so there shouldn't be more than two or three ingredients on the list of ingredients on your peanut butter.

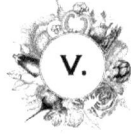

Chapter V.
Making Healthy Choices

Making healthy choices will improve health, promote a healthy BMI, increase energy, improve metabolism, and improve overall quality of life.

Reducing your intake of red meat to one serving each week is one step in the right direction once you have chosen to live a healthy lifestyle. I rarely eat pork or beef, but when I do, I look for lean cuts such as pork tenderloin, beef round, beef chuck, or sirloin.

Plan to eat fish two or three times a week, and be sure to select fish high in omega-3 fatty acids, such as salmon, trout, and tuna. On the other days, get most of your protein from organic chicken and lean turkey. Your poultry should be lean and skinless. Ask for white meat when possible since the dark meat usually has more fat. It is important to watch your portion sizes on meat for nutritional and health purposes.

> *On average, you should have two or three servings of protein each day.*

This serving recommendation varies or may change based on sex, health and fitness goals, or health status. Each serving should be about three or four ounces. When purchasing ground meat, look for meat that is at least 95 percent lean. Avoid processed meat such as bologna, hot dogs, and sausage. Processed meats may contain sodium nitrites and nitrates, which can form carcinogenic compounds, have very little nutritional value, and are completely bad for you. The next time you go to the ball park, skip the all-American hot dog!

There are many meatless sources of protein if you live a vegan lifestyle. Many people stand by the myth that we must eat meat for protein. This is not true at all. In fact, I recommend getting most of your macronutrients from nonanimal products when possible. I am not recommending that everyone become vegan—I am simply recommending that we consume less animal-based foods and more plant-based foods for better overall health and longevity.

A few examples of plant-based sources of protein are brown rice, quinoa, tofu, lentils, beans, green peas, broccoli, brussels sprouts, spinach, edamame, nuts, seeds, nut butters, and oatmeal. Many of the vegetables we eat contain protein, however most Americans are unaware of this fact. A serving of most plant-based foods contains fewer grams of protein per ounce than most meat contains per serving, but you can eat a higher volume of plant-based foods containing protein and get less calories and less fat than you would with a smaller serving of meat with similar amounts of protein per ounce of meat. For example, it would take more than eleven cups of broccoli (about 330 calories), to equal the amount of protein in one cup of grilled chicken (240 calories). Although you get a few more calories with eleven cups of broccoli, there is almost no fat, very little sodium, no cholesterol, and lots of nutrients. In addition, the broccoli will fill you up and last much longer than the cup of chicken. It would take most people a few hours or longer to eat eleven cups of broccoli, but most of us will finish a cup of chicken in a matter of minutes and may not feel completely satisfied.

Some studies suggest that dairy can aid in weight loss, specifically loss of belly fat.

> *As I continue to suggest, it is a good idea*
> *to limit your intake of dairy*
> *since it is an animal product.*
> *Choose low-fat or fat-free versions of dairy*
> *with no sugar added.*

Good sources of dairy are low-fat cottage cheese, organic low-fat greek yogurt, and skim or 1 percent milk. Personally, I don't eat a lot of dairy, mainly because I try to eat as little animal-based foods as possible. For several years I have been intentional about limiting my meat and dairy intake. I am not vegan, but the research on plant-based diets and the animal-farming industry was enough to convince me to reduce my intake at the very least.

Some fruit has more sugar than others, and some vegetables are starchier than others, so choose fruits and vegetables that are not too starchy. You can refer to an online glycemic-index scale to determine how your carbohydrates are ranked. If you are trying to lose weight, corn and peas probably shouldn't be your vegetable of choice since they are very starchy vegetables. Although corn and peas are nutritious, a better choice than processed food, and should be a part of your diet, they are not the best substitute for green leafy vegetables such as spinach, broccoli, and asparagus. Whole grain foods with high fiber content such as baked sweet potatoes, brown rice, and quinoa are the best choices, and don't forget to read your labels on your bread. Many people make the mistake of thinking a bread is good for you just because it says "whole wheat." If it says enriched it probably contains white flour and is possibly low in fiber. Aim for at least three grams of fiber per serving on your bread. One of the first ingredients should be whole grain. For breakfast cereals, choose one with fewer than six grams of sugar and at least five grams of fiber if you must have cereal. I recommend oatmeal as your first choice of cereal. If possible, choose steel cut oats. They are filling because it takes longer to digest them, and they are packed with fiber and whole grains. The only disadvantage that comes with steel cut oats is that they take much longer to cook than old-fashioned or quick oats.

> *Don't drink all of your calories!*
> *Alcohol and sugary beverages such as juice,*
> *sugary coffee drinks (lattes, Frappuccinos,*
> *or cappuccinos) contain a lot of calories and sugar*
> *and may prevent you from achieving*
> *your fitness and weight-loss goals.*

Although excessive amounts of caffeine can be unhealthy, a cup or two of coffee is not bad for you. Coffee becomes unhealthy when we start adding creamers and sweeteners. If you can't seem to enjoy your coffee black, there are a few semi healthy options, such as adding a tablespoon of unsweetened almond milk, and stevia. When using sweetener for your coffee, raw organic sugar cane, stevia, raw organic honey, or raw organic agave nectar are the best choices. Use a dash of cinnamon when sweetening your coffee, as this helps stabilize blood sugar and prevent blood-sugar spikes. Instead of using creamer in your coffee, try sticking to unsweetened almond milk or skim milk since they are lower in sugar and calories. The best drinks to have on a daily basis are unsweetened tea (green, black, or white with the same sweetening recommendations as coffee) and of course water.

> *Failing to drink enough water*
> *will result in dehydration, which causes the body*
> *to hold on to excess water and results*
> *in a higher number on the scale.*

Hydrate yourself, so your body will release the excess fluid and toxins on its own. Dehydration can also result in headaches and lack of energy, which can make it difficult to power through your workout. Exercising with an excruciating headache is extremely difficult, so be proactive and remain hydrated. There is absolutely *no* nutritional value in diet or regular soda. In fact, if you are going to drink an occasional soda you might as well drink a regular coke rather than diet. Remember that nature is better than science as it relates to our food supply, therefore artificial sweeteners found in diet sodas are not better for you than natural sweeteners. Diet soda is loaded with artificial sweeteners, and it contributes to cravings and weight gain. My recommendation is to avoid soda altogether. Adopt and practice a healthier lifestyle, including healthy eating habits, and commit to becoming educated on fitness and nutrition. Become more active, and make this your lifestyle versus something to do until you lose the excess weight. If adopting a healthy lifestyle is something you plan to do temporarily because you have a vacation coming up, before a special date arrives, or to fit into your skinny jeans or swimsuit by summer you will more than likely gain the weight back. You are at high risk for gaining the weight back and returning to an unhappy state because your mind-set is consistent with temporary goals and a temporary healthy lifestyle. Your new lifestyle should be a lifelong commitment so that you can maintain your results.

Remaining mindful of situations and specific environments that are likely to put you in the danger zone, are key for success. For example, restaurants while traveling, parties, celebrations, special events, and baby/bridal showers are all situations or settings in which we are at risk of overeating or making poor choices. Having an idea of what you plan to order prior to entering a restaurant is very helpful in remaining on track with making healthy choices. Choose lean protein such as turkey, grilled or baked fish, or grilled or baked chicken when ordering an entrée, while searching for options containing beans, rice, vegetables, and grains for healthy vegan options. Some restaurants offer bowls in which you can choose the ingredients for your entrée. Skip side dishes such as cheesy potatoes, fries, and creamed spinach if you are trying to lose weight. Baked potatoes, brown rice, and whole grains are the best choices for starches. Adding creamy sauces, butter, salt, and sugar to vegetables is typically not a good idea since it makes them fattening and unhealthy. Steamed broccoli, green beans, asparagus, spinach, or any green vegetable with no sauce are great choices for vegetables. There will be days or special occasions on which you plan to eat more than you typically do, or choose foods that aren't as healthy as the food you typically eat. Planning is key on these days that you are away from home and have less control over what is served.

Do your research, and find out if there are restaurants close to your job and home that have healthy items on their menu. Once you learn which restaurants have items consistent with your meal plan and goals, stick to those restaurants as your choices of places to eat at when you don't have time to make meals at home.

There will be times at which you feel pressured to indulge in unhealthy habits. For example, when staff at your office are serving donuts for breakfast or having a luncheon. It is okay for you to decline the donuts and not feel obligated to indulge. Choose dishes that are lower in calories, low in sugar, and free of artificial ingredients when attending showers and parties. Your coworkers will respect your healthy eating habits, and eventually you might influence some of them to adopt healthy habits. When choosing not to partake in an office luncheon, you should not completely remove yourself from the group for the sake of trying to stay on track with your fitness or weight-loss goals. Grab a bottle of water and a healthy snack, and enjoy interacting with your coworkers. Prior to arriving at a party or special event, eat a filling snack that includes protein, and drink a large glass of water so that the sweet and high-calorie treats will be less appealing. A small amount of fiber is also a good idea to help remain full between meals. Contribute a healthy dish when attending parties and events. This will ensure there is something healthy there for you to eat in case you get hungry and there are no other healthy dishes to choose from.

> *Socializing and having a good time does not have to involve overeating or sabotaging your health and fitness goals.*

Travel time and vacations are also very difficult when trying to maintain a healthy lifestyle. When I am going to be away from home for more than a few hours, I almost always pack a couple of snacks, such as granola bars, protein bars, boiled eggs, fruit, healthy meal-replacement shakes, and nuts. If you are going to be in a hotel, oatmeal packets are a good idea for breakfast because you can make them with the coffee maker simply by filling the coffee pot with water and mixing the hot water with the oatmeal. Eat plain oatmeal, and add your own ingredients, such as cinnamon, raisins, banana slices, or natural peanut butter, instead of using flavored oatmeal. This is filling and will keep you full until you are able to search for a healthy lunch. As I mentioned previously, meal replacement shakes are also a great choice for breakfast or lunch. If you need a good meal replacement shake contact me to order our shakes. We can have them shipped directly to you. Having lean protein and vegetables for dinner is the best choice. I don't recommend having starches after noon. If you need help with meal planning send an email and we will email your meal plan.

Protein bars can be a good addition to your meal plan, depending on your training regimen. When purchasing protein bars or granola bars, be sure to determine if you want it to serve as a protein supplement, meal replacement, or as a light snack. Review the nutritional facts and the ingredient list on the packaging prior to purchasing—this will help you to determine what type of bar to purchase. If your snack/protein bar is 250 calories or more, use it as a meal replacement rather than a snack (depending on weight, fitness goals, weight loss goals, daily caloric goal, etc.). There are a few snack bars that are low in sugar, does not contain trans fats, are low in calories and high in fiber, and are made with natural ingredients. Search for a protein-packed bar or a clean meal-replacement bar. Typically, the fewer ingredients they contain, the better they are for you. There are plenty of good protein bars on the market, and making your own is also an option.

Sometimes we think we are eating healthy food until we look at the ingredient list and learn that our "health food" is loaded with sugar, artificial ingredients, and chemicals. If you are a body builder, trying to pack on muscle, or on a twenty-five-hundred-calorie or more diet, a three-hundred-calorie granola bar or protein bar is going to be a snack for you rather than a meal. It would be a meal replacement for people who are trying to remain under fifteen hundred calories each day.

A major factor in making healthy choices and living a healthy lifestyle is being consistent. This means remaining active and staying on your meal plan when at home and when traveling. Most hotels have an on-site fitness center, so skipping your workout while away from home should not be an option. Schedule thirty minutes of exercise in the fitness center everyday while traveling. Taking a swim in the pool while at your hotel is also a great way to burn calories while away. Swimming is a low-impact way to burn some calories and will help you remain on track with living a healthy lifestyle while away from home.

> *The ultimate goal of most fitness and slimming programs is to increase the amount of lean-muscle mass and reduce body-fat percentage.*

That means burning fat and building muscle for a lean and toned look. It does not always mean losing weight. One pound of muscle weighs the same as one pound of fat, but muscle provides a much more attractive look. Very often trainers and fitness professionals observe clients who do not lose very much weight according to the scale, but their waist is smaller, their thighs and arms are more toned, their clothes become too large for them, and their overall build is leaner with a lower percentage of body fat. Although we live in a society where everyone wants to be thin, it is important to understand that skinny doesn't necessarily equate to good health.

Lean is healthy, but malnourished is not. We need a little bit of muscle to protect our bones, help with balance and stabilization, help fight disease, and to improve our metabolism. This becomes increasingly important as we age. There are many individuals who are naturally very thin and very healthy, and some who are a bit heavier and just as healthy. Focusing on achieving a healthy body-fat percentage, healthy eating habits, daily exercise, and living an overall healthy lifestyle are much more important than focusing on being skinny.

To battle obesity, you don't need to be an expert on fitness and nutrition, you don't need to starve yourself, you don't need a magic pill, and you don't have to spend all day in the gym. Educate yourself on sound nutrition, implement what you have learned into your daily life, incorporate a consistent fitness regimen into your daily routine, plan your meals carefully, and secure a support system to help achieve your health and fitness goals. Be sure to get your fitness and nutrition advice/education from a reputable and qualified professional. We live in a time where everyone is an "expert" at everything due to the Internet. Remember that the Internet is a wonderful resource, but you don't have to be a professional, an expert, or even have the correct information to have a YouTube channel, to "go live" with an informational recording on social media, or to sell a product. All it takes is hitting the record, post, or share button. There are many reputable health and fitness professionals on the Internet who provide good, sound fitness and nutrition advice, but make sure you check their credentials and/or experience prior to hiring them as your trainer, nutritionist, coach, or for other services. When searching for a professional, sometimes experience can be just as valuable as degrees, certifications, or licenses. As a person who has degrees, licenses, and certifications, I truly believe that if you are passionate enough about your profession, you will pursue the necessary credentials to become a reputable resource in your industry regardless of how experienced you are. Pursuing the necessary education, licenses, and certifications to acquire the necessary credentials to become a reputable professional is an indicator of an individual's commitment to their trade. This also demonstrates whether they have the personal discipline they are trying to instill in their clients, listeners, or readers.

> *Although there are many experienced individuals*
> *providing health and fitness services,*
> *it is important to seek advice and services from*
> *qualified, certified, and licensed professionals.*

This will reduce the risk of injury and ensure the best results from your fitness and nutrition program.

Fad diets typically require you to follow a low calorie diet with a very restricted food list. Your daily diet should be one that you can maintain long-term. Following an 800 calorie diet is not sustainable, and will usually result in short term results. Drastically reducing calories on these low calorie or restrictive diets can be detrimental to your metabolism. When metabolism is negatively impacted, your body stores excess calories as fat which is counterproductive if you have weight-loss goals. Eating the right foods, with the right portions, at the right time will help burn fat, build muscle, and/or lose weight.

16 SIMPLE STEPS
TO INCORPORATE INTO YOUR DAY
AND PROMOTE A HEALTHY LIFESTYLE

1. **Eat about five times** per day to improve metabolism and remain full between meals.

2. **Drink one glass of warm water** with the juice from one-half fresh lemon first thing in the morning, prior to starting your day. This helps with cleansing and detoxifying the body.

3. Plan to **get at least twenty - thirty minutes of cardiovascular exercise** in the morning before starting your day (fasted cardio is a good choice). You must make time in your schedule for exercise. Scheduling exercise ahead of time is helpful.

4. **Eat breakfast daily** within one hour of waking or right after your morning workout.

5. **Eat a combination of lean protein and complex carbohydrates** at each meal.

6. Do **eat small amounts of healthy fats daily** (nuts, olive oil, flaxseed oil, sunflower oil, walnut oil, safflower oil, avocado, olives, nuts, and seeds).

7. **Drink a minimum of sixty-four ounces of water** each day. Ideally half of your body weight in ounces is recommended, especially if you are active.

8. **Plan your meals when you plan your workout.** I recommend getting this done before you start your day. If you write down your meal plan before the day begins, you are more likely to stick to it. Make sure you have everything you need at home to prepare the meals you have planned. Check each item off the list as you eat them throughout the day. This will increase the chances of remaining on track. Everything you intend to be a success in your life should be planned and written down. There will be occasional curve balls thrown into your plans, but it is not impossible to recalculate or readjust your plan. You must consider your work schedule, family responsibilities, travel for business, and other responsibilities when planning in order to establish and maintain balance.

9. **Join an online fitness community.** This will allow you to share your struggles and successes with others who are interested in fitness and in living a healthy lifestyle. This also connects you to others who may support and encourage you during the hours that you are not at the gym or with your fitness buddies. It is easy to get off track with nutrition while at home with our families on the weekends, while on vacation as previously stated, or when spending time with friends and colleagues. In addition, if you have children, more than likely you have constant access to snacks that are not on your meal plan. It is important to remain in contact with others who motivate you and inspire you to remain on track with your goals. Remember that you can't do this alone. Most of us have tried to lose weight or get fit by ourselves many times and failed.

10. **Weigh and measure your food,** and *never* supersize your meals when you eat at restaurants. Supersizing your meals typically means you are supersizing your waist! In fact, refrain from eating

at an establishment that offers supersizing as an option altogether. That's usually not a place you should eat anyway, especially if you have weight-loss or fitness goals you are trying to accomplish.

11. **Read food labels.** Most food and beverages marketed as being healthy simply aren't healthy.

12. **Avoid going to all-you-can-eat buffets.** Eating at a buffet one to four times a year is plenty for this type of overindulgence, especially if you are trying to lose weight. Most people think they can go to a buffet without overeating. It is very difficult to track everything you are consuming at an all-you-can-eat buffet.

13. **Get excited about your goals!** Losing weight or getting in shape requires both physical and mental preparation. Instead of waiting for the perfect time, it is better to get into the mind-set now. There is never a perfect time to start your weight-loss journey or to plan to live a healthier lifestyle. Don't wait until tomorrow, don't wait until Monday, don't wait until after the holidays, don't wait until the New Year. Make it happen *today*!

14. **Avoid all-or-nothing thinking.** I call this "distorted" or "faulty" thinking. You don't have to give up everything at once in order to succeed. Making small lifestyle changes will help you remain consistent and on track with your goals over time.

15. **Make a commitment to yourself,** and share it with someone else for accountability. Be sure the person you share your plan/goals with is someone who cares about your health and well-being and will hold you accountable. Sharing your health and fitness goals with someone who does not take your goals

seriously is counterproductive and will more than likely create extra stress and conflict throughout your journey.

16. **Eat a little protein with every meal** and snack. It helps keep your blood sugar from spiking. Blood-sugar spikes result in hunger and cravings. Remember, protein also helps you remain satisfied between meals.

A Mediterranean-style diet can be instrumental in trying to give your metabolism a boost and is a proven way to ensure you are making healthy choices. This type of diet focuses on fresh fruits and vegetables, fish, poultry, legumes, grains, and olive oil. A lower-carb style of the Mediterranean diet is the best choice in rebooting your metabolism. According to research reported from Spain and Italy, low-carb Mediterranean meal plans triggered rapid fat loss and major improvements in overall health. To burn fat instead of carbs, eat fewer starches after lunch, fill up with good carbs like fibrous veggies paired with lean protein in the afternoon and evening, and drink eight to twelve ounces of water with each meal.

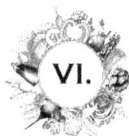

VI.

CHAPTER VI.

PORTION CONTROL

Controlling your portions is another important strategy in achieving your health and fitness goals. An adequate portion of meat for a single meal is three to five ounces, which is about the size of the palm of your hand. Choose lean cuts of meat rather than cuts with excess fat. Eating your meals slowly will help reduce the chances of overeating.

It is imperative that we redefine the word diet. In the United States we refer to a diet as a restrictive and unsatisfying way of eating in order to lose or maintain weight.

> *The true definition of diet is "a particular selection of food."*

In other words, your diet is simply the choices in food you make on a daily basis, whether the choices are good or bad. Keep a food journal for at least one week in order to determine whether your current diet is sufficient for your specific goals or whether it will inhibit your progress. It is highly likely that you will need to discuss your journal with a dietician or a certified nutrition specialist to determine if your diet is ideal for your goals.

Eating water-rich foods and lean protein daily and drinking two cups of green tea daily also helps curb appetite between meals and boosts metabolism. When we are satiated or full after each meal, we are more likely to maintain appropriate portions during each meal.

Having one or two cups of water, half an apple, and one hard-boiled egg or a handful of nuts will reduce your chances of overeating. This will provide you with complex carbohydrates, protein, and hydration, which will result in satiety.

OTHER PORTION - CONTROL STRATEGIES

1. **Refrain from feeling obligated to clean your plate**. Studies show that 54 percent of Americans eat until their plates are clean. Many of us were expected to do so as children and still feel the need to do so. Your mother will forgive you if refraining from cleaning your plate will save your life.

2. When eating at a restaurant, **stop eating once you are satisfied and no longer hungry**, rather than when you are full. Most restaurants serve meals that contain portions large enough to be divided into two meals. Divide your meals in half and place half of it in a takeout container prior to eating. This will help reduce the chances of overeating.

3. **Use smaller dishes.** It is important to make sure your plates are not oversized. We tend to eat more when eating from a larger plate or bowl.

4. **Reduce occurrences of mindless munching during meals.** Over 30 percent of people who eat at restaurants that serve unlimited bread or dinner rolls during meals have a hard time recalling the amount of bread they ate during their meal. If you tend to munch on dinner bread mindlessly as you wait on your meal, it is a good idea to have the bread removed from your table altogether, especially if you are trying to lose weight.

5. **Serve healthy foods family style.** In other words, sit the foods that you want your family to eat more of such as salads, fresh fruit, raw nuts, and vegetables within easy reach on the table or kitchen countertop.

6. **Think before you drink.** If you are drinking anything other than water, you might want to drink eight to twelve ounces of water first. This will ensure you have quenched your thirst first and you are not relying on juice, sports drinks, or other beverages to do what only water can do. If you are depending on a beverage that is high in calories or sugar to do what only water can do (satisfy thirst), you might find yourself drinking several grams of sugar and several calories before you find out you need water. Most drinks that are marketed as being healthy usually aren't. For hydration and overall health, pure water and an occasional cup of freshly brewed tea or coffee are the best choices. You can add fresh or frozen fruit to your water for extra flavor and nutrients.

7. **Avoid watching television while you eat.** Studies show that we are more likely to consume more calories if we are watching television while eating or snacking.

8. **Refrain from keeping dishes of candy** and unhealthy treats sitting around on the table at home or on your desk at work. You are more likely to overindulge if it is in your face all day.

9. If you are the "gatekeeper" or "overseer" of food in your house, use your power for good. This means **you are in charge of purchasing food and preparing food** at least 70 percent of the time, so make good choices.

There are several other strategies and tips for controlling portions, these are simply the basics.

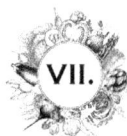

VII.

CHAPTER VII.

EATING TO LIVE

DISEASE - FIGHTING FOODS

When we think of diseases we fear the most, cancer is probably at the top of the list. There are several foods we can incorporate into our diet to help reduce the risk of developing cancer or other chronic illnesses.

Eating the right foods can have endless benefits.
Your daily diet can aid in weight loss,
help prevent disease, and give you more energy.

Women who eat sweet potatoes, bell peppers, carrots, spinach, tomatoes, and kale may reduce the risk of developing breast cancer by up to 20 percent. These power foods contain carotenoids, which are building blocks for vitamin A. Men and women both benefit significantly from carotenoids and vitamin A. Vitamin A regulates growth and death of cells. Eating foods rich in carotenoids and vitamin A can also act as antioxidants which can deter the oxidative stress that can trigger cancer growth. Garlic, fatty fish (such as salmon and mackerel), and berries may also help reduce the risk of developing breast cancer. Many of us have learned that food is the enemy as it relates to health, but the exact opposite is true. Food and nutrient intake play a major role in health and reducing the risk of disease. In order for the food we eat to enhance our life, prevent disease, help achieve a healthy weight, and improve our overall health status we must have an adequate amount of nutrients, a healthy balance of each food group, balanced caloric intake, self-control, portion control, nutrient-dense food, moderation, and variety.

FOODS THAT HAVE THE ABILITY TO IMPROVE OVERALL HEALTH AND FIGHT DISEASE

1. **Bananas** protect against ulcers because they are rich in compounds that protect digestive health by destroying bacteria in the stomach lining.

2. **Flaxseeds** are rich in fiber and make us feel full, which decreases the amount of daily calories consumed. They are great for our digestive system and can help with constipation.

3. **Apples** are full of fiber, help reduce appetite, and can assist in stabilizing blood sugar. Apples are also rich in phenolic phytochemicals, which are antioxidants that protect neurons in the brain from oxidative stress. This can aid in reducing the risk of Alzheimer's and other degenerative conditions. Do not peel apples or discard skin. Eat the entire apple (except the core) to fill up on pectin, a soluble fiber that helps feel full longer and stabilizes blood glucose levels. A study conducted by University of Iowa researchers discovered Ursolic acid, a unique compound in apple peels increases lean muscle mass. These effects have

proven to increase calorie burn, ward off weight gain and fatty liver disease, and stabilize blood sugar.

4. **Berries** can reduce a woman's risk of heart attack by 34 percent, simply by eating them at least three times a week, according to Eric Rimm, an associate professor of epidemiology and nutrition at Harvard School of Public Health. Rimm reports strawberries and blueberries are loaded with anthocyanins, compounds that might help lower blood pressure by keeping arteries elastic.

5. **Cabbage** may cut risk of breast cancer by 40 percent. Cruciferous veggies such as cabbage and broccoli contain indoles, which are phytonutrients that affect precancerous cells, reducing breast-cancer risk by 40 percent. Indoles also help your liver break down harmful estrogens according to the Natural Hormone Institute in Jacksonville, Florida.

6. **Whole grains** reduce the risk of cervical cancer. Women who eat foods that are 100 percent whole grain such as brown rice, barley, and oats are less likely to get cervical cancer than women who eat excessive amounts of starch made with white flour. Whole grains are rich in vitamins that have proven to stop the growth of abnormal cervical cells, including B vitamins, selenium, and vitamin E. Try three servings per day.

7. **Beets** increase muscle blood flow and nitric oxide production. Nitric oxide is a gas released by the inner lining of blood vessels that is essential in regulating blood flow and blood pressure. This could improve overall aerobic performance. Beets are also found to be effective in helping the liver function properly.

8. **Fish** contains disease-fighting omega-3s, which may help protect the heart, and contributes to the prevention of cardiovascular disease. We have been told for years that omega-3 fatty acids are good for the heart and the cardiovascular system. Fatty fish such as herring, lake trout, mackerel, salmon, sardines, and albacore tuna are all high in omega-3 fatty acids. Some fish contain dangerous levels of environmental contaminants such as mercury and dioxins. This is typically the case in larger, older, predatory fish and marine mammals. The FDA advises children and pregnant women to avoid eating fish with the highest levels of mercury contamination (king mackerel, shark, swordfish, and tilefish). It is recommended that children and pregnant women choose canned light tuna, salmon, pollack, and catfish over other types of fish.

9. **Spinach** is a very popular green vegetable due to its superfood status. Scientists at Harvard Medical School suggest individuals who eat dark leafy green vegetables such as spinach are less likely to develop cataracts. This is mainly due to the lutein found in this vegetable. Lutein is a carotenoid that prevents the breakdown of proteins in the lenses of the eye. Spinach is a great source of iron (very beneficial to vegetarians). Iron is beneficial for red blood cells that fuel our muscles with oxygen for energy. Spinach is high in fiber, high in antioxidants, anti-inflammatory, strengthens the immune system, promotes strong bones, and is low in calories while high in nutrients. Add spinach to salads, wraps, sandwiches, and omelets, or steam and eat them as a side dish with meals. Spinach is also good when added to marinara sauce and served over whole grain pasta, grilled chicken, or added to meatloaf.

10. **Cocoa** is high in antioxidants and delivers potent benefits to the cardiovascular system, brain, and immune system. This healthy substance is good for your mood as well.

Plant-based foods contain naturally occurring compounds called phytonutrients.

> *Phytonutrients have the ability to protect against heart disease and cancer, and aid in weight loss.*

Genistein, quercetin, and resveratrol are all phytonutrients that aid in improved health and weight loss. Resveratrol is a natural compound found in grapes, mulberries, peanuts, red wine, and cocoa powder. Resveratrol has been found to protect against cancer and cardiovascular disease by acting as an antioxidant and anti-inflammatory. Quercetin is a phytonutrient found in apples and tea and is used medically to treat capillary fragility. Genistein is an isoflavone found in a number of plants such as soybeans and chickpeas that acts as an antioxidant and counteracts damaging effects of free radicals in tissues. Dr. Rayalam, a researcher at the University of Georgia in Athens, found that the synergy among genistein, resveratrol, and quercetin can stop new fat cells from developing, prevent maturing of existing fat cells, and even cause fat-filled cells to self-destruct.

FOODS THAT AID IN WEIGHT LOSS

1. **Grapefruit** has proven to burn and help release fat. They are a great addition to your daily diet. Grapefruit may help you feel full when eaten before a meal due to the soluble fiber they have in them. Organic grapefruit is a great choice, but it is not necessary since you will not be consuming the peel or outer layer as you will with apples.

2. **Cinnamon** is a great way to help regulate blood sugar. When your blood sugar is regulated, your appetite is kept under control. Intense food and sugar cravings are sometimes the result of unstable blood sugar. Cinnamon can be added to coffee, tea, yogurt, or fruit daily.

3. **Mushrooms** help to stabilize blood sugar. When used in place of meat, it is possible to shed pounds more rapidly. Mushrooms are high in fiber, which is good for controlling the appetite. Because mushrooms aid in keeping blood sugar in check, they help prevent food and sugar cravings and help to avoid fatigue and afternoon energy crashes that accompany unsteady blood sugar.

4. **Avocado** is a very popular health food. The monounsaturated fats in avocado boost the body's production of hormones that speed up metabolism. A study from UCLA found that when people ate a burger with avocado, their arteries remained more flexible for hours afterward, compared to eating burgers alone. Research also suggests BMI and waist size among people who eat avocado are typically smaller than those who do not eat it.

5. **Vinegar** contains acetic acid, which slows the passage of food from the stomach into the small intestine so you stay full longer. Take one tablespoon three times a day to stimulate metabolism and to aid in cleansing of the internal organs. Raw organic apple-cider vinegar has more health benefits than other types of vinegar. Vinegar can also prevent or reduce blood-sugar spikes that occur after eating a meal containing refined carbs. Calories are no concern with vinegar, which is why using this rather than salad dressing on salads is a smart choice.

6. **Green tea** can speed up your metabolism and helps control hunger. Organic green tea is the best choice. Try drinking one cup in the morning and one cup in the afternoon. Research has found that catechins in this drink can increase the burning of belly fat for fuel during exercise.

7. **Do not to add sweetener** to your tea or coffee. If you must have sweetener, use raw organic sugar cane, raw honey, or stevia. These are all better for you than artificial sweeteners or refined sugars. Read the ingredients to make sure your stevia does not include any additives and that it is 100 percent stevia.

8. **Artificial sweeteners can contain potentially harmful chemicals** that can slow down your metabolism. Refined sugars are horrible for your blood-sugar levels and contribute to obesity. Remember, it is always best to consume foods, condiments, and drinks that are closest to their natural state with as little processing as possible,so artificial sweeteners are not a good idea.

9. **Organic yerba mate tea** may help increase mental focus and mental alertness, increase energy, and decrease appetite. Try drinking a cup of warm tea after meals to aid in digestion of

food and to prevent clogging of the arteries. Recent research suggests cold beverages after meals may contribute to clogging of the arteries.

10. **Hot peppers** contain capsaicin, which may help speed up metabolism and can aid in decreasing appetite. Add hot peppers to salads, wraps, stir fry, and other healthy dishes. Salsa that contains hot peppers is also a good choice to add to omelets, burritos, wraps, and so forth.

11. **Greek yogurt** has twice the protein as other types of yogurt. Protein takes longer to leave the stomach and keeps you full longer. The body burns more calories when digesting protein than it does with carbs.

12. **Quinoa** is packed with whole grains, protein, and fiber. Quinoa also has iron, zinc, selenium, and vitamin E. Mix in veggies, nuts, or lean protein to get variety and extra nutrients.

13. **Raw veggies** help satisfy the desire to crunch, so pick up a plate of them instead of potato chips. They are also low in calories and have a high water content, which can help us feel full between meals.

14. **Pears, apples, and berries** are high in fiber and water to help us feel full longer.

15. **Watermelon** contains lycopene and vitamins A and C. Lycopene is a very powerful antioxidant that may help protect cells in the body from damage. Since watermelon is full of water, it takes up more room in the belly than many other types of fruit and helps us stay full longer. Although watermelon is good for you, it

contains quite a bit of natural sugar. If you are trying to avoid blood-sugar spikes or trying to lose weight, you should avoid overindulging in this particular fruit, just as you would with most fruit.

16. **Beans** are an excellent addition to your diet. It is a veggie that contains protein and a ton of fiber. There are many different types of beans to choose from. According to Joseph Colella, MD, a bariatric surgeon at Magee-Women's Hospital in Pittsburg, your body has to work to breakdown the bean to get through the fiber, so you are actually expending energy to digest them. He also reports the protein in beans and legumes makes us feel satisfied. This results in eating fewer calories and smaller portions.

17. **Nuts** can be a great snack between meals to curb appetite, but you must be careful because they are high in calories. Just a handful a day will do. Nuts are high in healthy monounsaturated fat, which is a necessary fat for your body to function optimally.

18. **Eggs** keep us full longer than starch. One egg packs about seventy-five calories and seven grams of protein. Our bodies burn more calories digesting a high-protein food such as eggs than with a carb-heavy breakfast such as cereal, toast, or pancakes.

19. **Summer squash** (zucchini and yellow squash) can help with weight loss because it is what some may call a negative-calorie food. This means they burn more energy/calories during digestion than they actually contain. I don't necessarily agree with the negative-calorie food theory, but there are several foods that are very low in calories and very nutritious and that keep you full

and aid in weight loss. Other low-calorie foods are arugula, asparagus, broccoli, broth, brussels sprouts, cabbage, lettuce, beets, cauliflower, coffee (black), tea, grapefruit, mushrooms, tomatoes, turnips, watercress, zucchini, spinach, lemons, limes, kale, garlic, peppers, onions, pumpkin, radishes, fennel, celery, berries, and carrots.

CHOOSING THE RIGHT FOOD FOR YOUR AGE

There are important foods we should eat throughout each decade of our lives to maintain healthy metabolism for life.

Our twenties is a good time to build bones by eating foods rich in calcium such as leafy green vegetables and low-fat dairy.

Our metabolism starts to decline at a rate of about 2 percent per decade after age thirty. Keep your metabolism fired up by spicing up your meals with peppers. Jalapeños and cayenne pepper are both good choices.

Due to hormonal changes that occur in our forties, it becomes harder to get rid of belly fat. Eat more plant-based foods such as produce, nuts, edamame, and tofu.

During our fifties and beyond is a great time to increase our fiber intake with fruits, vegetables, and whole grains. These foods can help cleanse our arteries of fatty deposits, which can help prevent and/or fight diabetes and keep us feeling full.

SIX FOODS AND BEVERAGES TO AVOID

1. **MSG** is a flavor enhancer and preservative that contributes to weight gain.

2. **Nitrates** are found in processed meats such as hot dogs and cause hormonal imbalances that lead to cravings and ultimately weight gain

3. **Fast food** is typically of poor quality and contains very little nutritional value. There are unbelievable amounts of hidden sugar, sodium, and unhealthy fats in most of the fast food we eat.

4. **Trans fats** are a type of unsaturated fat that is uncommon in nature but became commonly produced from vegetable fats for use in margarine, snack food, packaged baked goods, and fast food starting in the 1950s. Any food containing this type of fat should be avoided at all costs.

5. **High-fructose** corn syrup is found in at least 70 percent of prepackaged food. This sweetener can damage the body's appetite-suppressing hormones, which can make losing weight impossible. Since food manufacturers began using HFCS in the 1960s, the obesity problem in the United States has continued to rise. HFCS can also be found in foods that are considered "healthy foods" such as some varieties of granola bars, breads, and low-fat yogurt. The easiest way to avoid HFCS is to stay away from processed foods and sugary drinks. We must also read ingredient lists prior to purchasing food to ensure we are aware of what we are putting in our bodies.

6. **Artificial sweeteners** are also an item to refrain from consuming since they contain chemicals, are unhealthy, and make it difficult to lose weight.

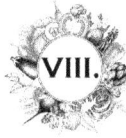

CHAPTER VIII.

SUPPLEMENTATION

The type of supplements you use are strongly dependent upon your goals. Fish oil and a multivitamin are a good place to start for everyone. However, women should consider adding calcium and vitamin D. For individuals who desire to gain lean muscle mass, a high-quality protein powder, (there are several on the market), and branched chain amino acids (BCAAs) are two of the most basic and effective supplements for muscle gain.

A high-quality meal-replacement shake can aid in weight loss for some individuals. Do your research and learn about the ingredients in your shake. Some meal-replacement shakes are marketed as "weight loss" shakes but are full of sugar, artificial ingredients, and chemicals.

There are numerous supplements on the market, but not all supplements are necessary for every individual.

> *A consultation with a professional*
> *who is an expert on supplements*
> *will help you determine*
> *the right supplements for you.*

It is always best to try to achieve as much of your nutritional needs, vitamins, and minerals from a well-balanced diet. Just because someone else takes a particular supplement, it does not mean you should. The supplement market is not well regulated, so you face the risk of taking supplements that may not work or may be harmful to your health. Remember to check with your doctor before starting a new supplement regimen.

Keep in mind that certain foods or supplements can be hazardous if taken with certain prescriptions or over-the-counter medications. *Always* read warning labels on medication and supplements, and consult with your physician and/or pharmacist before taking new supplements.

We should use dietary supplements to enhance or add to our daily dietary intake, rather than as a permanent substitute for natural whole food.

Many Americans do not have an adequate amount of nutrients in their daily diet due to avoiding specific food groups, lack of variety in diet, eating only one meal per day, consuming excessive amounts of junk food, and economic limitations.

SIX OF THE MOST NECESSARY SUPPLEMENTS

1. **Vitamin D** may protect against heart disease, and many researchers believe that it guards against cardiovascular risk factors such as diabetes and inflammation. Vitamin D also reduces the risk of multiple sclerosis, stroke, colon cancer, breast cancer, and type 2 diabetes. The best way to boost vitamin D levels is through sun exposure. During winter months, a vitamin D supplement may be necessary to assist in getting daily recommended amount due to lack of exposure to sunshine. Higher levels of vitamin D have been linked to greater muscle strength and bone health, and very important for calcium metabolism and absorption. Athletes who play indoor sports are more likely to be deficient in vitamin D than athletes who play outdoor sports. Do not exceed recommended doses of vitamin D due to potential risk of calcification of arteries and brain, nausea, and other potentially harmful side effects.

2. **Fish oil** can reduce your risk of osteoarthritis by 50 percent, according to British researchers. Fish oil may also reduce breast-cancer risk by 30 percent according to Scientists at the Fred Hutchinson Cancer Research Center. Danish researchers also report a woman's risk of developing heart disease is significantly reduced when getting plenty of omega-3s.

3. **Whey protein** promotes metabolic health by improving blood-sugar levels, insulin regulation, and appetite control. It also reduces inflammation and increases lean muscle mass.

4. **Magnesium** may help reduce the risk of cancer, helps control inflammation, and helps regulate many other bodily functions.

5. **B - complex** may help you remain energized throughout the day and helps convert food into energy.

6. **Multivitamins** are good for people who do not have a well-balanced diet and body builders, and it is very important for active individuals. Multivitamins promote the presence of essential nutrients necessary for metabolic reactions and processes.

Talk to your physician about whether you should implement a multivitamin or any of the aforementioned supplements into your daily supplement regimen.

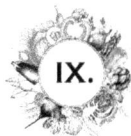

IX.

CHAPTER IX.

SUGAR IS THE CULPRIT

Sugar has a significant impact on weight gain. Your blood-sugar levels have a direct impact on weight gain and weight loss. When your blood sugar is around 120, you are in the weight-gain zone, at 90 you are in the fat-burning zone, and at 60 you will more than likely experience constant hunger, cravings, and fatigue. Pasta, crackers, cereal, bread, desserts, candy, and other sweet treats raise your blood-sugar levels. It is important to be selective about the type of carbohydrates we consume to keep blood-sugar levels at a healthy level. Sprouted grain bread, rice, spelt, quinoa, millet, sweet potatoes, fruits, and vegetables are good carbs that reduce the chances of blood-sugar spikes.

> *Skip the sugar!*
> *Eating sugary foods such as desserts and candy*
> *can spike your insulin levels,*
> *which releases signals to your body to store fat.*

In the past our society focused on low-fat or fat-free diets, but unless the fat we consume is trans fat, sugar should be more of a concern than fat.

Sugar consumption is linked to weight gain for many reasons. Sugar tends to be concentrated in packaged foods and fast food, which results in more calories. When we eat high-carb meals or sugary snacks, our glucose levels increase. Excessive glucose is toxic and causes insulin levels to increase in order to get the glucose out of the bloodstream and into the cells. Insulin is the hormone that regulates our metabolism and energy use and is secreted by the pancreas. If we didn't have insulin, or if it wasn't functioning properly, blood glucose would reach toxic levels in our bodies. When insulin levels are chronically elevated, a great deal of the energy in our bloodstream gets deposited in fat cells and stored. When we develop insulin resistance due to excess fructose consumption, our bodies have a difficult time accessing stored fat and the brain thinks it is hungry. This results in eating more, which contributes to weight gain. Studies show that sugar causes dopamine activity in the reward centers of the brain, similar to the effect of other drugs such as cocaine. Sugar is very addictive. This explains why individuals that often have strong cravings for sugar find it very difficult to reduce their consumption of sugar, regardless of negative consequences such as weight gain.

It is important to remain very careful about selecting refined and artificial sweeteners, since the research on them is unclear and controversial. Agave nectar comes from the Mexican agave plant and is a decent choice. It is much sweeter than sugar so you will only use small amounts of it. Agave also contains small amounts of iron, calcium, potassium, and magnesium, which are good for refueling your workout. Try to stick with raw organic agave when possible. You will still get blood-sugar spikes from agave but not as much as you do with refined white sugar. Although agave is a slightly better choice than regular refined granulated sugar, it still isn't the best choice.

Artificial sweeteners are just that, artificial and fake. Please do not trust them or use them.

> *Plan to eat foods that are as close*
> *to their natural state as possible.*

Artificial sweeteners have been linked to obesity and illnesses such as cancer. These findings are still inconclusive and controversial. However, the most important thing to remember in our food choices is to choose whole, natural, and unrefined/unprocessed foods.

Stevia is a healthy option for a sweetener. It is important to read the ingredients because some stevia products on the market are not 100 percent pure stevia. You will find that some have artificial sweeteners added. If it's 100 percent pure stevia, it is your best choice between the other sweeteners I have listed.

Raw organic sugar cane will still cause blood-sugar spikes, but it is not as refined as white sugar, so it is a better choice than white refined sugar. The body processes all sugars the same, and doesn't necessarily notice the difference between raw sugar, refined sugar, or natural sugar. Although this is true, it is still a good idea to remain choosy about the types of sugar you use. As previously stated, nature is always the better choice when it comes to our food supply, so pick items that are closest to their natural state.

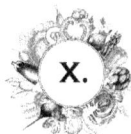

CHAPTER X.

HOW TO DRESS FOR YOUR BODY TYPE

An apple-shaped individual typically carries most of his or her weight in the waist or upper body and has slimmer hips, while a pear-shaped individual typically carries most of his or her weight around the hip with a smaller waist. There are many ways to complement our shapes simply by choosing the right clothing for our body type.

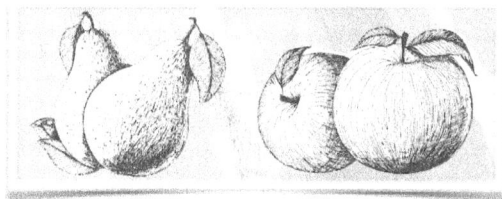

MEN

Apple-shaped men should avoid pants with a flat front and go for slacks with pleats in the front. Shirts should not be tucked in, but if the occasion calls for a nice shirt please tuck your shirt in! Wearing a blazer is a good idea for apple-shaped men, and vests with no jacket should be avoided.

Pear-shaped men should try to avoid skinny jeans or tight-fitting pants.

WOMEN

You have an apple shape when you tend to carry your weight around the stomach, have a larger bust size, and no defined waist. Many women start to develop an apple shape after forty, when they start to experience symptoms of perimenopause. Many people with an apple shape tend to try wearing loose clothing to cover up or hide their apple shape, which is not a good idea. To create the best silhouette with an apple shape it is a good idea to create an illusion of a waist, highlight cleavage, and create vertical lines. This creates a long and lean silhouette. Ruching is a good choice for tops on an apple shape. A dark V-neck top with a ruched center seam disguises a bulge in the midsection. This gives the illusion of curves and conceals a belly bulge. A ruffled V-neck that connects to the vertical seam helps draw the eye inward and up and down, which creates a longer leaner torso. Apple-shaped women usually have very shapely legs, so wearing lighter and fitted pants with a darker ruched top can draw the eye down away from the middle to create an attractive silhouette.

The best bottoms for an apple shape are skirts that have zippers on the side. It is important to make sure that any pleats in the skirt begin below the belly to avoid adding extra volume around the belly. Pencil skirts work very well for this body type, but be sure to keep them at knee length.

An apple shape looks best in jeans that are straight or flared. Pants with a high waist will help to create a nice silhouette. Make sure your pants do not cling to your stomach or thighs unless you are planning to create the long and lean silhouette with vertical lines as I stated earlier. Avoid pleats! Get slacks or pants that have zippers on the side to avoid adding any extra bulk in the front.

Since you draw a lot of attention to the top part of your body, make sure your bras are of good quality and fit very well. Going into a bra shop that specializes in bras to get measured and fitted is a good idea. Tops should cover the entire belly area and end just below the hip bone. Shirts on an apple-shape look best when they are tight just beneath the breast area and then flare out. Shirts with patterns tend to look good on an apple shape because they flatter and camouflage. Try finding tops with a thicker texture to avoid fabric that clings to the body. Overall, make sure you choose tops that highlight the slimmest point, which is usually just below the bust area. Make sure your tops provide enough room for the belly but aren't too wide in the midsection.

Dresses should have a waistline just below the bust, and jackets can help to create a nice silhouette when worn over tops. Make sure your jackets define your waistline and that they fit your shoulders perfectly. When shopping for jackets, be sure to get the right-size jacket for your shoulders rather than your belly. If you can't close the jacket, you can use a scarf to fill the gap, but it is a good idea to shop for jackets that you can close and fits your shoulders if possible. Jackets that have a nice V shape at the top look great with an apple shape.

Having a tie or belt in your slimmest area is a great choice, as it hides the belly and highlights the waist. You don't have to tie it at your natural waist and can go higher if necessary.

In addition, longer tops and jackets that fit closely to the body can be worn with leggings and skinny jeans. Make sure shirts are not too short, and layering with a cardigan or a long sleeveless vest is a good idea.

GARMENTS AND CLOTHING TO AVOID
WITH AN APPLE SHAPE

An individual with an apple shape should avoid everything in one solid color. Try mixing colors and textures or using several layers in different colors to create vertical lines. Avoid clingy shirts, high necklines, bulky pants with lots of pockets and zippers in front, puffy coats and jackets, and large shapeless garments that hide the waist or have no vertical layers.

A pear shape is the most common figure for women. This means that the widest part of the body is below the waist in the hip area. You can be thin, heavy, tall, or short and have a pear shape. If you are a pear shape, the goal is to elongate your shape so that you look less bottom-heavy. This means you have to balance your hips and shoulders while showing off your beautiful curves. With a pear shape, you have to accentuate your upper body with things such as fashionable scarves around your neck to take the focus off of your bottom half. Wearing darker garments on your lower half such as dark pants or a dark knee-length skirt is a good idea. You don't have to wear black or dark colors on your lower half all of the time, but make sure you wear solid colors and that your skirt or pants are darker than your top. Wearing prints, fun colors, or detail around the neck will draw the attention away from the hip area. Avoid wearing tops that end at your hips, since they will draw attention to that area.

A pear-shaped individual should stick with flat front pants and avoid pleats, side pockets, wide belts, and anything that might add bulk to the hip area. If you wear a belted dress, ensure the belt sits higher than your waistline rather than at the hips. Wearing a top gathered around the belly hides the tummy if necessary.

A pear-shaped individual should wear pants that have a flare on the bottom to draw the eye away from the hip. Avoid capris or tapered pants if you have a pear shape because they draw attention to the hips. Wear jackets that end past your hips rather than at the hips. A long jacket or blazer creates a long lean line and covers the hip area. Wearing long necklaces are also a great choice for pear-shaped individuals. This fills the neckline, which adds to the lengthening of the upper body.

If you are pear shaped, you want to show off your shoulders by wearing off-the-shoulder tops that expose one or both of the shoulders. These tops attract attention to the upper body and steer the eyes away from your hips. Keeping it simple on the bottom allows room to play with accessories and tops. Pear-shaped individuals should fill their wardrobe with skirts and pants that fit well and then play with trendy colors and prints for tops. Nice earrings, scarfs, and necklaces will help draw the eye up to your most amazing feature, your face! Pear-shaped individuals should choose material like wool slacks and denim because they flatter a pear shape. Avoid tight knits on the bottom since they cling to the body and accentuate width.

A ruffled dress with ruffled sleeves can be a good a choice for a pear-shaped woman. The texture and width of the sleeves draw attention to the top of the body and makes shoulders look more broad. The broader look on the ruffled shoulders make hips look smaller.

Curvy women are just as beautiful as women without curves, so if you are a curvy woman who prefers to show off those beautiful hips, then no need to make any wardrobe changes. Choosing a wardrobe to draw less attention to your shape or to accentuate your shape are both personal choices.

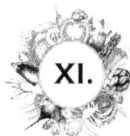

XI.

Chapter XI.

Training

Research has proven that exercising in the morning on an empty stomach can burn up to 20 percent more fat. I personally don't recommend my clients perform strength training on an empty stomach after fasting overnight, but "fasted cardio" can be quite effective. While sleeping overnight, the body is fasting for several hours, so the body is forced to burn stored fat for fuel when exercising in the morning. You have a few options regarding training and nutrition in the morning. Fasted cardio is when you have a cardio training session first thing in the morning prior to eating your first meal of the day. It has proven to be a very effective fat burning strategy.

> *If you plan to have a strength training session in the morning, it is a good idea to have a shake, smoothie, egg whites and spinach, or any healthy light snack before your training session.*

I do not recommend a heavy meal prior to training at any time, regardless of whether your training session will consist of cardio or strength training. Have a balanced meal consisting of complex carbs and protein within an hour after each training session.

A protein shake, meal-replacement shake, or smoothie is a good idea if you don't have immediate access to a healthy meal. Smoothies sometimes contain too much sugar, so don't go overboard with adding fruit. Your smoothing will be more nutritious if you make your own with fresh produce, ice, and unsweetened milk rather than buying premade smoothies

You can optimize metabolism and build lean muscle mass by mixing cardio exercise with strength training. A good way to start is three days of strength training and two days of cardio, three days of cardio and three days of strength training, or four days of strength and two days of cardio. Your training regimen will depend on your goals. Many fitness professionals will have you perform more cardio exercises than weight training, and some will have you perform more weight training than cardio. You may even find that some trainers only use strength training and believe that cardio is unnecessary. I personally recommend both cardiovascular training and strength training because they are both equally important. Cardio is important for overall cardiovascular health and for reducing body weight.

> *In addition, there is nothing like the natural high from the endorphins released after a nice long run or a cardio-intense training session.*
> *This is a natural antidepressant!*

Neither approach to training that I mentioned is an incorrect approach, but if you do your research, you will find that strength training produces the best results for reducing body-fat percentage and transforming your physique. Regardless of which training approach you take, please take one day off each week. You will get much better results if you allow adequate recovery time for each muscle group between training sessions. An intense cardiovascular workout can decrease strength and muscular endurance, so it is a good idea to get your strength training done first when doing cardio and strength training on the same day.

> *If you are a beginner,*
> *single sets are a great way to start.*

This would entail one set of each exercise. Start out with eight to twelve repetitions per exercise. Focus on increasing your number of sets (multiple sets, giant sets, supersets), and increasing the weight over time. Another effective training strategy is drop sets. This means you will perform a set until you reach muscle failure, then remove a small percentage of the load before continuing with the set with no rest until you run the rack (you have run out of weights) or reach muscle failure. For example, bicep curls starting out with the heaviest weight you can handle while maintaining good form. You would aim for eight to twelve or until you reach muscle failure, immediately reduce your weight, and continue with the reduced weight for the same number of reps or until reaching muscle failure, and then reducing the weight again and performing the same amount of reps or until you reach muscle failure. There is no rest between sets on drop sets. Most athletes do not use drop sets since their goals usually consist of gaining strength, power, and speed without the bulk. Body builders are mostly concerned with cosmetic improvements such as increasing muscle size (hypertrophy) rather than athletic performance. This is one of the reasons body builders prefer drop sets. Pyramid training is very similar, except you can increase or decrease weight with each set. With pyramid sets, you don't have to perform your set until you reach muscle failure.

Your trainer will help you learn more about these particular approaches to training and help you implement them into your training regimen if necessary.

An individual with a goal to build mass should add supersets, drop sets, pyramid training, and multiple sets to their routine. You have the option of doing a split routine, in which you only work certain muscle groups on certain days. I recommend this style of training simply because it allows sufficient recovery time, and you get the opportunity to give the necessary time and attention to training each muscle group-for example, chest, shoulders, and triceps on Monday, legs and abs on Wednesday, and back and biceps on Friday. You can also perform a total-body training session in which you work each of the aforementioned muscle groups on the same day. I recommend split-routine training, with an occasional total-body session.

> *Muscles are broken down during your training sessions, so it is necessary to allow the muscles an adequate amount of time to recover between training sessions and remain on track with nutrition, sleep, and hydration.*

These are all a very important part of the process body transformation and recovery process. Weight training is the best way to replace unwanted fat with lean muscle mass and to achieve the shape or physique we desire. For women who have no curves, weight training can help achieve curves in the right places. For example, squats can help achieve more curves in the hip area and create nice shapely glutes. Regular weight training also slims the waist, hence giving a nice shapely silhouette. Our metabolism improves as we build more lean muscle mass, therefore helping us burn more calories hours after our training session has ended. A post-workout supplement or a protein powder with muscle-recovery properties is very helpful in reducing soreness, building lean muscle mass, and enhancing recovery. Talk to your trainer about recommendations for post-workout or recovery formulas.

High-intensity interval training (HIIT) is very effective for losing weight and increasing cardiovascular endurance. The muscle you build during strength training helps your body burn more calories at rest. HIIT training combined with weight training builds strength, improves endurance, and reduces body-fat percentage. HIIT training involves intervals of exercises at a high level of intensity for a period, followed by a brief rest time before performing another interval of the same exercise or of a different exercise. Try adding HIIT training to your weekly fitness routine to accelerate your results. If you are in need of HIIT training programs contact me for programs you can do at home or on the go. We also offer HIIT at Club Exhilaration. Your trainer can also develop a HIIT training regimen for you.

> *Stretching is a very important part of your workout because it improves range of motion and reduces the risk of an injury.*

Certain types of stretching should be limited before certain types of exercise. The *Journal of Human Kinetics* reports recent studies have shown that excessive static stretching before weight training decreases muscle endurance, strength, and power. Completing a five- to ten-minute warm-up consisting of light cardio and dynamic stretching before strength training is a much better idea than excessive static stretching.

There are many barriers to exercise. Most Americans report if they had more time, more energy, and fewer obligations outside of the gym they would be more active. The truth is that when we have more time, we find other things to do rather than adding daily exercise to our schedule. Failing to exercise regularly usually results in ongoing fatigue, and makes it difficult to commit to other healthy choices such as maintaining a healthy diet. Over time we pack on pounds until we decide it's time to make changes. We find time and energy to do the things that we want to do, or things that are important to us in life, such as social media. Some of the very people who report they do not have enough time in their day to exercise for thirty minutes spend well over a couple of hours a day on social media sites, watching television, texting, and talking on the phone. Some excuses for not training regularly are legitimate, but typically we are simply talking ourselves out of exercising.

> *The key to making exercise a habit is scheduling it,*
> *setting an alarm, and consistently doing it*
> *on demand, just like we do everything else.*

For example, we set our alarms to wake up for work each day. As a result, we consistently wake up and get into our daily routine. We get our children to practice, games, concerts, classes, and recitals on time because it has become habit, and it is on our schedule. When we schedule these activities, we know that we have to do them at a certain time and on a specific day, so we do them without question or debate. Having the same strategy with our daily training session should be no different.

If you find that you are too tired to exercise, take into consideration that exercise or regular physical activity can improve or increase energy level. Start out by committing to a full week of exercise, and you will experience a significant difference in your energy level. After that first week, maintain a training regimen in which you train for thirty minutes to an hour for four or five days a week. Most people think exercise will decrease energy level since you are expending energy, but it has the opposite effect. Having an accountability partner or workout buddy will help adhere to your commitment to remain active, especially when you work full-time, have gone back to school, and/or have a family. That buddy/partner will be there to push you when you say you are too busy or too tired or are trying to skip out on your workout.

A couple of very common and unacceptable excuses for not engaging in daily exercise is not wanting to mess up a hairstyle, or not having the time to redo hair and makeup. It takes less than ten minutes to touch up hair and makeup. If you have a hairdo that prevents you from exercising, you might want to reevaluate your style. If you are unhealthy, overweight, and miserable, how much joy will that great hairstyle bring you? We are typically happier when we are satisfied with what we see when we look in the mirror, get a clean bill of health when visiting the doctor, have energy, and feel confident in our physical appearance. I know plenty of people with great hair, the latest fashion, expensive toys, and very well put together but not healthy due to lifestyle. Wouldn't all of that be more enjoyable if we were physically healthy and in shape? I love to get my hair done, in fact I change it very often. My hairstylist is very well aware that I must have a style that will not interfere with my training regimen. Hair, fashion, style, and looking great are important but not more important than our health. Hair is temporary and can be altered at any time. In fact, most of us will lose it sooner than we want to. The rest of your body will be around much longer than your hair, so our physical health should be a priority. Invest in makeup remover wipes to remove makeup before training. After your workout, cleanse face/ remove sweat, and reapply makeup if necessary.

> *There are several other benefits to exercise such as its natural appetite-suppressing effects.*

Studies have found that if you exercise at a moderate to vigorous level of intensity, a shift in hormones may aide in suppressing the appetite post-workout. This will help refrain from indulging in counterproductive overeating after your workout. Your post workout meal should be carefully planned out and consist of balanced nutrition geared toward refueling. A protein shake, or lean protein paired with whole grains and vegetables are all good choices for post workout meals.

Athletes sometimes follow intense training programs in their quest for better performance without adequate rest. This can result in overtraining. Overtraining is an imbalance between training and recovery. Although there is no single indicator of overtraining, some symptoms are decreased performance, injuries, elevated cortisol, depression, frequent illness, elevated resting heart rate, and muscle damage. Since hard work is necessary for improving fitness level, overworking your body for long periods results in elevated cortisol levels, failure, and breakdown. Be sure to listen to your body, and take a day off once a week. If you have been training at a vigorous and ongoing basis for several months and you're not getting the results you are seeking, this may also be an indication that your body needs a break. I don't recommend taking more than a couple of days off after several months of intense training, however a week off may be the answer to pushing through your plateau. Remember this may only be necessary if you have been training at a very intense level for several months, your body is showing signs of distress, and you aren't getting any results. During your week off, try walking, yoga, and light resistance exercises. During this week refrain from engaging in strenuous exercise, and stay on track with nutrition, sleep, and hydration. It may also be a good time to implement a slight detox consisting of no sugar (including fruit), no starch (including tortillas, brown rice, potatoes, quinoa), and no oil. Stick to lean protein, fresh vegetables, water, and green tea.

AN EXAMPLE OF A GOOD MEAL PLAN FOR THIS WEEK

1. **Breakfast:** a spinach, mushroom, and onion omelet (one whole egg and one or two egg whites)

2. **Morning snack:** half cucumber sliced sprinkled with apple-cider vinegar, and one cup freshly brewed organic green tea

3. **Lunch:** grilled-chicken salad (three ounces grilled or baked chicken, one or two cups spinach, romaine, or spring mix, one-fourth cup red onion, and no cream based dressing)

4. **Afternoon snack:** other half of cucumber with raw apple-cider vinegar and one cup freshly brewed organic green tea

5. **Dinner:** chicken and broccoli stir fry (three ounces baked or grilled chicken and one or two cups broccoli depending on daily calorie goal, one-fourth cup green onion, and one-half cup sliced mushrooms). I recommend using organic chicken when possible.

If you want to go a step further, try going meatless during your detox/recovery week. This would mean refraining from adding meat to your salads and stir fry. Increase your portion of veggies by up to one cup when refraining from eating meat. This will ensure you are satisfied after your meals. Mushrooms are a wonderful substitute for meat.

> *Portions during meals are always dependent on each individual's weight, goals, health status, and doctor's recommendations.*

Implementing such a detox is simply an option for flushing out the digestive track and stabilizing blood sugar, and is not necessary during your recovery week. I do not recommend trying this detox more than twice each calendar year, mainly because I do not recommend removing fresh fruits and whole grains from your daily diet for long periods. Fresh fruit and whole grains have necessary nutrients for fighting disease and for optimal health. It is completely acceptable to remove meat from your diet for long periods of time. Always consult with your physician before implementing any changes in your daily diet or supplement intake or when beginning a new fitness program.

Other options when facing a plateau are changing up your workout routine. Our bodies adjust to our fitness routine if we fail to change things up a bit. Muscle confusion is very effective in pushing past a plateau and achieving optimal results. Hiring a personal trainer can help you push past your plateau. A very large percentage of people who start a fitness program or a weight-loss program will quit before they get to the point where they are seeing results.

SOME OF THE MISTAKES PEOPLE MAKE

- poor planning;
- ignoring small victories;
- getting on a diet to lose weight for a single event;
- all-or-nothing mind-set;
- trying to do it alone;
- not allowing any time for fun or a social life;
- expecting quick results; and
- extreme/fad dieting

As previously stated, there are many physical and emotional health factors positively affected by exercise and by living a healthy lifestyle such as emotion and mood, quality of life, self-esteem, social activity, cognitive functioning, and sleep. In addition, exercise promotes longevity so hit the gym, hit the pavement, push play, or whatever your routine of breaking a sweat and burning calories is. You must get in the habit of doing this every day in order to reap the benefits.

DEVELOPING A GREAT PLAYLIST

Whether you are running, walking, strength training, using home fitness programs, or at the gym, motivating music is an absolute must. My favorite training songs have gotten me across the finish line many times. Think about the songs that give you energy, make you want to move, or make you feel you can conquer the world when you hear them. Those are the songs you should consider adding to your playlist. If your music sounds like good music to listen to when trying to relax, it is probably not good training music. Most people need upbeat music.

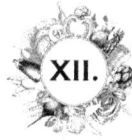

CHAPTER XII.

THE EMOTIONAL SIDE OF OBESITY

Weight loss, weight gain, or any struggle with our physical appearance is just as much of an emotional struggle as it is a physical battle. This battle can be even more emotionally challenging for someone who struggles with an addictive personality. Someone with an addictive personality is at high risk for becoming addicted to one thing after another.

For example, a person with an addictive personality may find that he or she has a food addiction, and may find that he or she eats when sad, mad, excited, and so forth. You may have heard this referred to as "emotional eating." This promotes weight gain or at the very least makes it difficult to lose weight.

An addictive personality refers to a set of personality traits that predispose a person to addictions.

Addictive behaviors are defined by the repetitive, excessive use of pleasurable activities to cope with internal conflict that is difficult to manage. Unmanageable stress and pressure are also factors.

It is suggested that there are common personality traits among people with varying addictions. People with addictive personalities are at a higher risk of becoming addicted to gambling, food, work, exercise, tobacco, drugs and/or alcohol, or becoming codependent. For example, if you are trying to lose weight and have been successful at giving up your addiction to food, you may be at a high risk for substituting another addiction for the food addiction. This explains why you might see a person who has been successful at weight loss become addicted to smoking, exercising excessively, or pick up some other habit.

Some might ask how being addicted to exercise can be a bad thing? Typically, exercise is 100 percent healthy and positive, but there are times in which excessive exercise can be harmful. Many people believe that the more they exercise, the better their results will be. This isn't necessarily true.

> *Excessive exercise without giving your body enough time to properly recover can force cortisol levels to remain elevated for long periods of time, which in turn will hinder your results and increase risk for injury.*

Overtraining combined with poor sleep habits, poor hydration, failure to properly supplement post-workout, and poor nutrition combined is a recipe for fatigue and injury. Another example of the potential for excessive exercise to have a negative impact on your life is when an individual is reaping the physical benefits of excessive training but his or her relationship with family is in trouble due to family time taking the backseat to training. Sometimes a person can get so focused on their goals that they fail to prioritize their life and responsibilities properly. If a husband and wife both work during the day, and one of them is at the gym for 3 hours every evening after work, this could cause tension in the relationship since the evening hours are the only hours the couple have to spend time together. Sometimes this can feel similar to an affair to the spouse at home. This typically doesn't become problematic unless it has occurred for several months and the couple isn't spending much time together at home or outside of the home.

While athletes are training for a competition or a big event, they are going to spend more time training than usual.

> *For the average person, an hour a day is sufficient, and anything more than two hours can be excessive.*

Some examples and signs that your training regimen is excessive are, training results in deterioration of physical or emotional health, does not promote improved quality of life, or interferes with family time. Depending on what your fitness goals are, fitness level, and the type of training you are implementing, thirty minutes a day may be sufficient. Your fitness level, goals, and other obligations will help to determine an adequate training prescription.

There are several other ways that an addictive personality can make it difficult to live a healthy lifestyle. Replacing a food addiction with excessive shopping or gambling is somewhat common. Many people like to find things to do in order to keep busy rather than sitting around with idle time. For most people who have gained control of their life by getting healthy, idle time equated to extra snacking or other bad habits in their past. In addition, most people who lose a significant amount of weight often find themselves shopping for new clothing to complement their new physique. This could contribute to financial problems if it becomes excessive, which in turn would have a negative impact on emotional health. A negative impact on emotional health would perpetuate the habit of emotional eating and ultimately hinder progress and goals.

Having an addictive personality can create a perpetual or revolving door of unhealthy and self-destructive habits and prevent an individual from living a healthy lifestyle. If you find that you are on a roller coaster of unhealthy behaviors and can't seem to break bad habits, talk to a professional about developing a plan that works for you. Finding balance is important in order to avoid getting involved with new unhealthy habits or returning to old unhealthy habits.

Other emotional aspects of health and fitness are discrimination and self-image. Unfortunately, being overweight can have a negative impact on how others see us and how we see ourselves, while being physically fit has many benefits, including our career status. Studies have shown that being overweight can hinder a person from moving up the corporate ladder or from getting a promotion at work. People tend to treat others who are thin or physically fit more pleasantly than they treat people who aren't. This is ridiculous, unkind, and very wrong, but it has been proven to be true. Most of this treatment is based on assumptions and stereotypes. For example, many people believe that an overweight person eats too often and too much, is lazy, and is overweight by choice. These are all untrue for many individuals who struggle with weight problems.

Most overweight clients I have worked with don't eat enough, have dieted excessively to try to lose weight, and have tried exercise but have a hard time finding the right fitness program to accommodate their fitness level.

> *Human beings treating other humans unfairly based on their physical appearance is unacceptable. However, this happens often.*

The unfair treatment and discrimination that an overweight individual often experiences can result in depression, poor self-image, lack of confidence, and feelings of anger and/or resentment.

When or if your weight begins to have a negative impact on your emotional or mental health, please seek help from a therapist to address the emotional distress, a personal trainer to help you get motivated and on track with a fitness regimen, a dietician to help you develop a well-rounded meal plan, and a physician to assess your overall physical health. Some individuals might only need to hire a trainer, some might only need a doctor to check overall health status and possibly prescribe medication, some may only need a counselor to address mental and emotional health, others may only need a dietician to educate them on proper eating habits, and some may need to seek help from more than one of the listed professionals in order to gain control of their physical and emotional health. Please remember whatever your needs are there is help!

FINDING YOUR "HAPPY WEIGHT"

When it comes to weight, it is easy to become obsessive or self-critical. Studies have shown that we tend to overestimate the size of our bodies by 15 percent or more, especially women. The main problem with this is that trying to achieve an unrealistic weight can negatively impact self-image and overall happiness. A study conducted by Janet Polivy, a psychology professor at the University of Toronto, revealed trying to achieve an unrealistic weight that is too low makes an individual feel like a failure when he or she can't achieve or maintain the extreme measures needed to force his or her body below a healthy weight. The study also revealed that subjects also felt like a failure when they reached the unrealistic weight, and couldn't maintain it.

Other studies have shown that when subjects stop trying to achieve an overly thin body, they are happier, they feel more attractive, and they become more assertive and more sociable. This allows people to gain more control over their quality of life.

We have to accept genetics to some degree, but this does not mean that you will inevitably end up overweight, simply because a large percentage of your family members are overweight. It also does not mean that if most of your family has no defined muscle tone, you can't achieve it. You might have to work harder than someone who has a naturally muscular build to build muscle, or you might have to work harder to lose weight or remain at a healthy weight than someone who has a naturally lean build, however, it is achievable.

> *Be consistent, add variety to your workout, get enough rest, remain hydrated, supplement properly, and maintain a diet that complements your goals. Never compare yourself to someone else because we are all very different genetically.*

Striving for a particular size or weight is fine, but please remember it is much more important to be healthy than to be a size two. It is 100 percent possible to be physically healthy while maintaining a healthy body weight for most individuals, therefore there is no need to rely on unhealthy tactics to lose weight. Take your time, do it right, get guidance from someone qualified to help, and develop the right habits to live a healthy lifestyle. Work toward improving physical health, spiritual health, and mental health so that your overall quality of life is improved rather than just improving certain areas life. Keep in mind that this is a lifelong journey rather than a temporary one. In other words achieving your health and fitness goals will be more of a marathon than a sprint. Once you get there, you have to practice the same habits to maintain your results as you did to achieve the results in the first place. There is no magic pill, wrap, or drink to get you there overnight. You have to do the work every single day. Don't forget nutrition is eighty percent of your work. You can't "out exercise" a bad diet, and what you put in your mouth this month you will wear on your body next month. You have all of the tools to make it happen!

You have planned to get healthy, tried to accomplish your health and fitness goals, started and stopped numerous times, and continue to wait for the perfect time to get back on track.

> *Yesterday you said you would get started tomorrow.*
> *Today is the day,*
> *so make it happen today.*

XIII.

CHAPTER XIII.

RECIPES

SPINACH - AND - TURKEY ROLLUPS

INGREDIENTS

2 tsp. honey mustard
a dash of nutmeg
8 slices of turkey breast
1 cup baby spinach
½ medium red bell pepper seeded and cut into thin strips
4 cheese string sticks

PREPARATION

1. In a small bowl, stir honey mustard and nutmeg together. Carefully spread mixture evenly over turkey slices.
2. Divide spinach among turkey slices, allowing leaves to extend beyond the turkey. Top with pepper strips and cheese.
3. Starting at an edge of turkey and cheese, roll up each turkey slice.

Calories: 40; fat: 1 g; sat. fat: 1 g; sodium: 220 mg; carbs: 1 g; protein: 5 g (per serving).

Makes eight servings

BREAKFAST TACOS

INGREDIENTS

2 small corn tortillas

1 tbsp. salsa

2 tbsp. reduced-fat shredded sharp cheddar cheese

1 dash cooking spray

½ cup egg substitute

PREPARATION

1. Top tortillas with salsa and cheese. Heat in microwave about 25 seconds.
2. Meanwhile, coat skillet with cooking spray. Heat over medium heat, add eggs, and cook. Stir until eggs are cooked through (around 2 minutes).
3. Divide scrambled eggs between tacos and enjoy.

Calories: 153; sat. fat: 1 g; sodium: 453 mg; total fat: 2 g; carbs: 15 g; protein: 17 g, cholesterol: 3 mg (per serving).

Add spinach, onions, mushrooms, cayenne pepper, or avocado for added taste and nutrients.

APPLE - CINNAMON WAFFLE

INGREDIENTS

1 whole grain waffle
¾ cup unsweetened applesauce
1 tbsp. chopped walnuts
a sprinkle of ground cinnamon

PREPARATION

Toast the waffle, and top it with applesauce, walnuts, and cinnamon.

Calories: 250; protein: 3 g; carbs: 43 g; fiber: 6 g; fat: 9 g; sodium: 200 mg (per serving).

GUAC - AND - TURKEY ROLL

INGREDIENTS

1 medium whole wheat tortilla
2 slices deli turkey
¼ avocado, peeled and sliced

PREPARATION

Top tortilla with turkey and avocado, and roll it up. Easy!

Calories: 231; protein: 13 g; carbs: 35 g; fiber: 6 g; fat: 9 g; sodium: 679 mg (per serving).

EASY OVERNIGHT OATMEAL

INGREDIENTS

½ cup old-fashioned oats
1 cup unsweetened vanilla almond milk
½ cup blueberries
2 tbsp. sliced almonds

PREPARATION

Combine all ingredients in a bowl and refrigerate overnight. Oatmeal will be ready to eat in the morning!

Calories: 250; protein: 11 g; carbs: 43 g; fiber: 8 g; fat: 15 g; sodium: 181 mg (per serving).

GRILLED LEMON CHICKEN

INGREDIENTS

2–3 tbsp. lemon juice

1 tbsp. white vinegar

2 tbsp. chopped fresh dill

2 tbsp. chopped fresh basil

1 tbsp. honey

1 tbsp. Dijon mustard

¼ tsp. black pepper

¾ tsp. salt

¼ cup extra virgin olive oil

6 boneless skinless chicken-breast halves (2–3 lbs.) pounded slightly

1 lemon, thinly sliced

⅓ cup pitted kalamata olives, halved

PREPARATION

1. For dressing, whisk together lemon juice, vinegar, dill, basil, honey, pepper, salt, and mustard. Slowly pour in oil and whisk.

2. Place chicken in a large resealable bag. Add ⅓ cup of the dressing and half the lemon slices. Seal bag; refrigerate 2 hours, turning at least once. Save remaining dressing, stirring in olives and remaining lemon slices.

3. Discard marinade and grill chicken over medium-hot coals for about 6 minutes per side.

4. Place chicken on a platter and drizzle with dressing; season with a dash of salt to taste.

    Calories: 347; protein: 44 g; carbs: 7 g; fat: 15 g fat; fiber: 0 g (per serving).

    Makes 6 servings

TRAIL MIX

Get sandwich bags and make your own rather than purchasing prepackaged trail mix. Most of the prepackaged options for trail mix are loaded with sugar, mainly because most of the dried fruit in them are coated with large amounts of sugar. Make sure the nuts you use are raw and don't contain sugar or salt. Make sure your dried fruit does not contain added sugar. Remember that nuts contain healthy fat but eaten in excess can contribute to weight gain or slow down weight loss results. I don't recommend eating nuts everyday due to high calorie count, but eaten in moderation, they can be a healthy snack to keep you satisfied between meals.

INGREDIENTS

1 oz. raw nuts (almonds, walnuts, or pistachios are good choices)
1 oz. raisins, dried cranberries, or any dried fruit that does not contain added sugar

Calories: depending on the type of nuts or dry fruit

KALE CHIPS
TOTAL TIME: 25 MINUTES

INGREDIENTS
1 large bunch kale, tough stems removed, leaves torn into pieces
(about 16 cups; see note at the end)
1 tbsp. extra virgin olive oil
¼ tsp. sea salt

PREPARATION
1. Preheat oven to 400°F. If kale is wet, pat dry with a clean kitchen towel (paper towels usually don't cut it). Be sure dry thoroughly - otherwise your chips might end up soggier and less crunchy. Transfer kale to a large bowl and drizzle with oil and then sprinkle with seat salt. Massage the oil and salt onto the leaves to evenly coat. Fill two large baking sheets with a single layer, making sure the leaves do not overlap.
2. Bake until most leaves are crisp, switching the pans back to front and top to bottom halfway through, 8 to 12 minutes total. (If baking a batch on just one sheet, start checking after 8 minutes to prevent burning.)
Store in an airtight container at room temperature for up to two days. Note: Choose organic kale when possible. Nonorganic can have high pesticide residue.

Calories: 110; fat: 5 g (sat. fat: 1 g, mono: 3 g); cholesterol: 0 mg; carbs: 16 g; added sugars: 0 g; protein: 5 g; fiber: 6 g; sodium: 210 mg; potassium: 642 mg (per serving).
Makes 4 servings, about 2 cups each

Turkey - and - Avocado Rollups

Ingredients

6 slices of all natural turkey breast
½ avocado sliced

Preparation

1. Lay turkey breast flat on a plate.
2. Lay a slice of avocado on top of each piece of turkey.
3. Roll each slice of turkey with avocado in it. You can also use low fat cheese, but the avocado keeps this snack a bit more on the clean side.

Pack them up in a storage container and eat 2 rollups for a snack.

Calories: 175, protein: 10 g; carbs: 11g; fat: 11g; sugar: 2g.

Makes 6 rollups; serving size is 2 rollups

BAKED APPLE WITH ALMOND AND PEAR FILLING

INGREDIENTS

1 large organic apple, cored and halved

2 tsp. reduced-fat cream cheese, divided

1 small organic pear, cored and diced in small pieces

½ tsp. light brown sugar

1/8 tsp. ground cinnamon

2 tbsp. chopped almonds, divided

3 tbsp. water

PREPARATION

1. Preheat oven to 350°F.
2. Slice apple in half. Scoop out some of the apple flesh from each half with a spoon or small ice cream scoop.
3. Dab 1 teaspoon of cream cheese inside each half.
4. Toss the diced pear with brown sugar and cinnamon.
5. Spoon pear filling into each apple half. Sprinkle almonds on pear filling, while pressing down to keep them in place.
6. Place apple halves in a baking dish and add water to the dish. Cover and bake for 30 minutes, then baste with juices. Bake uncovered for another 10 minutes, or until almonds are roasted.

Calories: 136; total fat: 3 g; sat. fat: 1 g; cholesterol: 3 mg; sodium: 16 mg; carbs: 28 g; fiber: 5 g; protein: 2 g (per serving). Makes 2 servings

ENJOY!

RESOURCES

Baile, C. A., Yang, J. Y., Rayalam, S., Hartzell, D. L., Lai, C. Y., Andersen, C., Della-Fera, M. A., 2011 "Effect of Resveratrol on Fat Mobilization."

Centers for Disease Control. "2008 Physical Activity Guidelines for Americans." 2015 health.gov

Williams, Jon. "How Many Calories Does Digestion Use Up?" 2014 livestrong.com

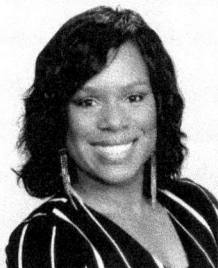

ABOUT THE AUTHOR

Carmel Brown is a Certified Personal Trainer, a Certified Fitness and Nutrition Specialist, and Co-Owner of Club Exhilaration Fitness Center where she and her husband help their clients and members transform their bodies and their lives.

Carmel specializes in one on one training and coaching, small group training, individual and group counseling and coaching, and meal planning. In addition, Carmel is a public speaker as she speaks, trains, and coaches at various events while helping her audience begin and maintain a healthy lifestyle, transform their bodies, improve mental health and emotional well-being, and ultimately improve their quality of life.

Carmel is also a Licensed Counselor which qualifies her to help clients push through mental and physical barriers to achieve a healthy body, healthy mind, and a transformed life.

For health and fitness coaching or counseling
visit the author website at:
WWW. CARMELBROWNCOUNSELING.COM

Make it happen today!

www.ingramcontent.com/pod-product-compliance
Lightning Source LLC
Chambersburg PA
CBHW050528280326
41933CB00011B/1510